National Theatre

Spring 2010 Season

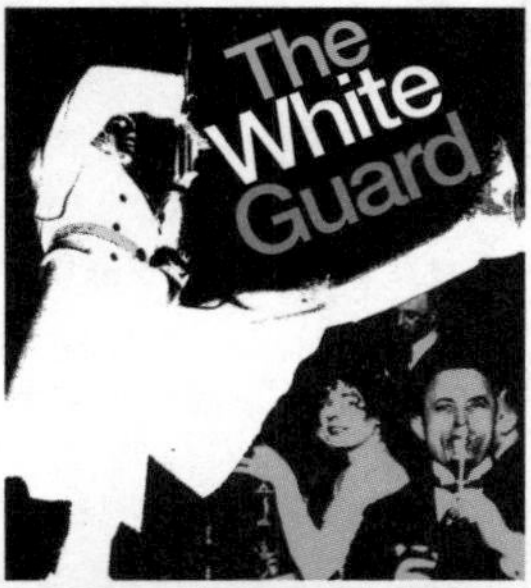

The White Guard
by Mikhail Bulgakov

A major new staging of Bulgakov's rarely-performed masterpiece, set amidst the near-farcical chaos of the Russian civil war.

From 15 March

Supported by American Express

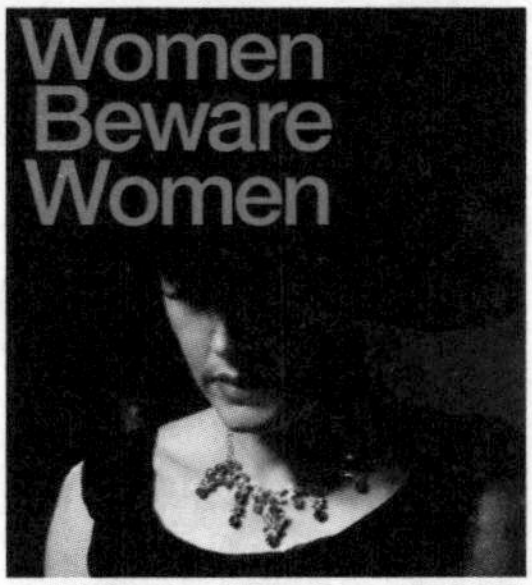

Women Beware Women
by Thomas Middleton

Travelex £10 Tickets

Corruption will not go unpunished in Middleton's blackly funny, fast and ferocious tragedy.

From 20 April

TRAVELEX £10 TICKETS
Sponsored by Travelex worldwide money

Media Partner THE TIMES

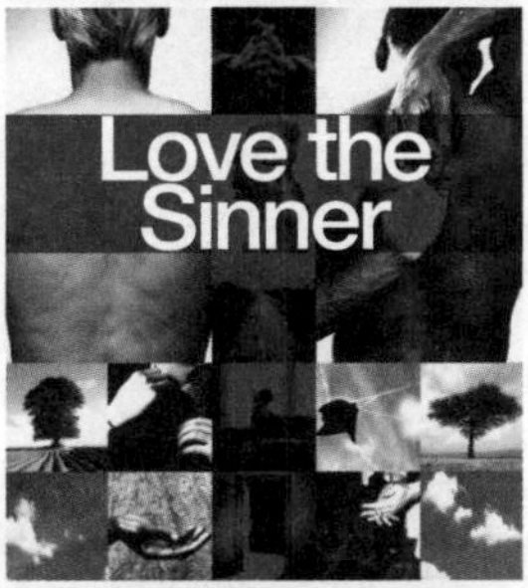

Love the Sinner
a new play by Drew Pautz

A tense and provocative new play, which unfolds against a backdrop of fierce debate within the Christian church.

From 4 May

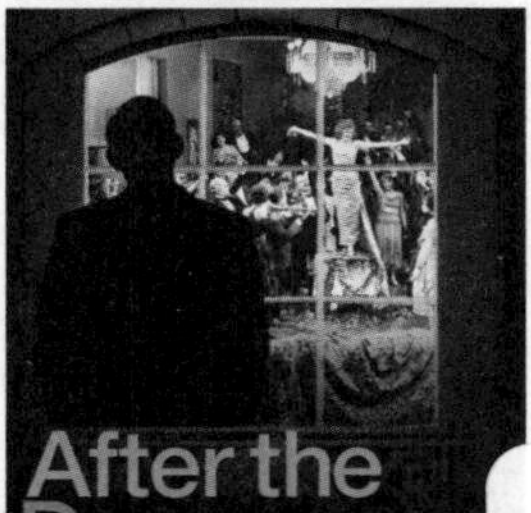

After the Dance
by Terence Rattigan

Rattigan's devastating play offers a subtle, witty unmasking of the hedonistic 1920s generation.

From 1 June

Supported by ARTS COUNCIL ENGLAND

020 7452

nationaltheatre.org.uk

GRANTA

12 Addison Avenue, London W11 4QR
e-mail editorial@granta.com
To subscribe go to www.granta.com
Or call 845-267-3031 (toll-free 866-438-6150) in the United States, 020 8955 7011 in the United Kingdom

ISSUE 110

In the United States, *Granta* is published in association with Grove/Atlantic Inc, 841 Broadway, 4th Floor, New York, NY 10003, and distributed by PGW. All editorial queries should be addressed to the London office.

Granta USPS 000-508 is published four times per year (March, June, September and December) by *Granta* 12 Addison Avenue, London W11 4QR, United Kingdom at the annual subscription rate of £34.95 and $45.99.

Airfreight and mailing in the USA by Agent named Air Business, C/O Worldnet Shipping USA Inc., 149-35 177th Street, Jamaica, New York, NY 11434. Periodicals postage paid at Jamaica NY 11431.

US POSTMASTER: Send address changes to *Granta*, PO Box 359 Congers, NY 10920-0359.

Granta is printed and bound in Italy by Legoprint. This magazine is printed on paper that fulfils the criteria for 'Paper for permanent document' according to ISO 9706 and the American Library Standard ANSI/NIZO Z39.48-1992 and has been certified by the Forest Stewardship Council (FSC). *Granta* is indexed in the American Humanities Index.

ISBN 978-1-905881-16-1

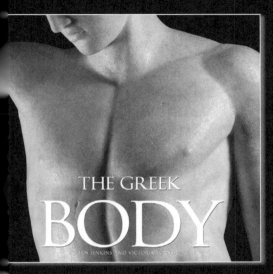

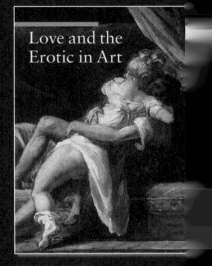

CONTENTS

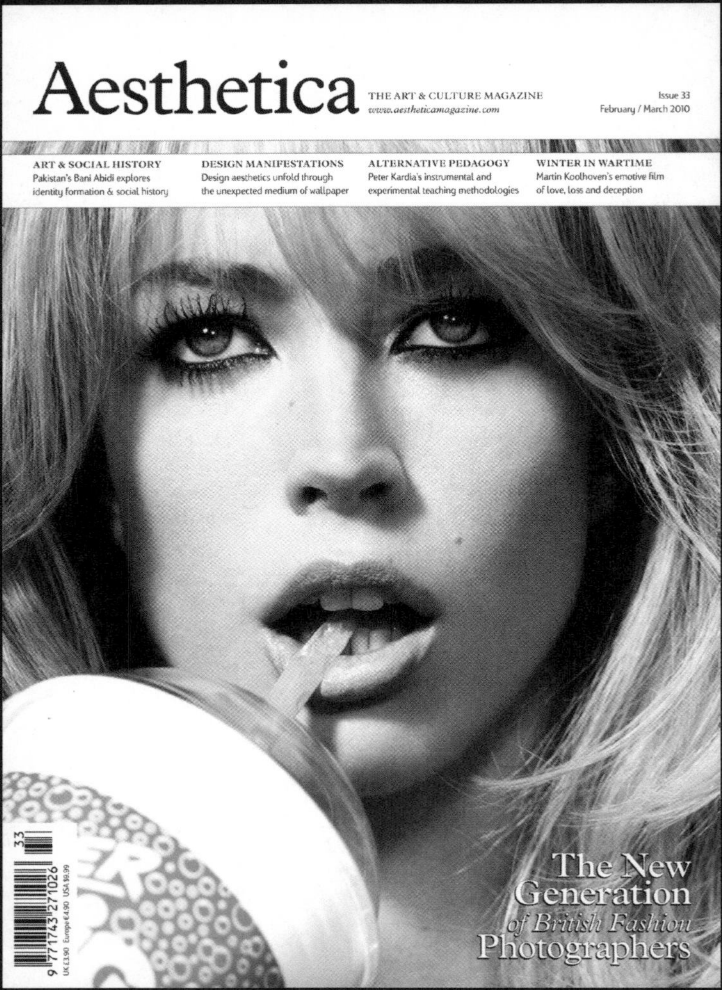
Aesthetica
THE ART & CULTURE MAGAZINE
www.aestheticamagazine.com
Issue 33
February / March 2010
ART & SOCIAL HISTORY
Pakistan's Bani Abidi explores identity formation & social history
DESIGN MANIFESTATIONS
Design aesthetics unfold through the unexpected medium of wallpaper
ALTERNATIVE PEDAGOGY
Peter Kardia's instrumental and experimental teaching methodologies
WINTER IN WARTIME
Martin Koolhoven's emotive film of love, loss and deception
The New Generation of British Fashion Photographers
UK £3.90 Europe €4.90 USA $9.99

THE UNWRITEABLE

Mark Doty

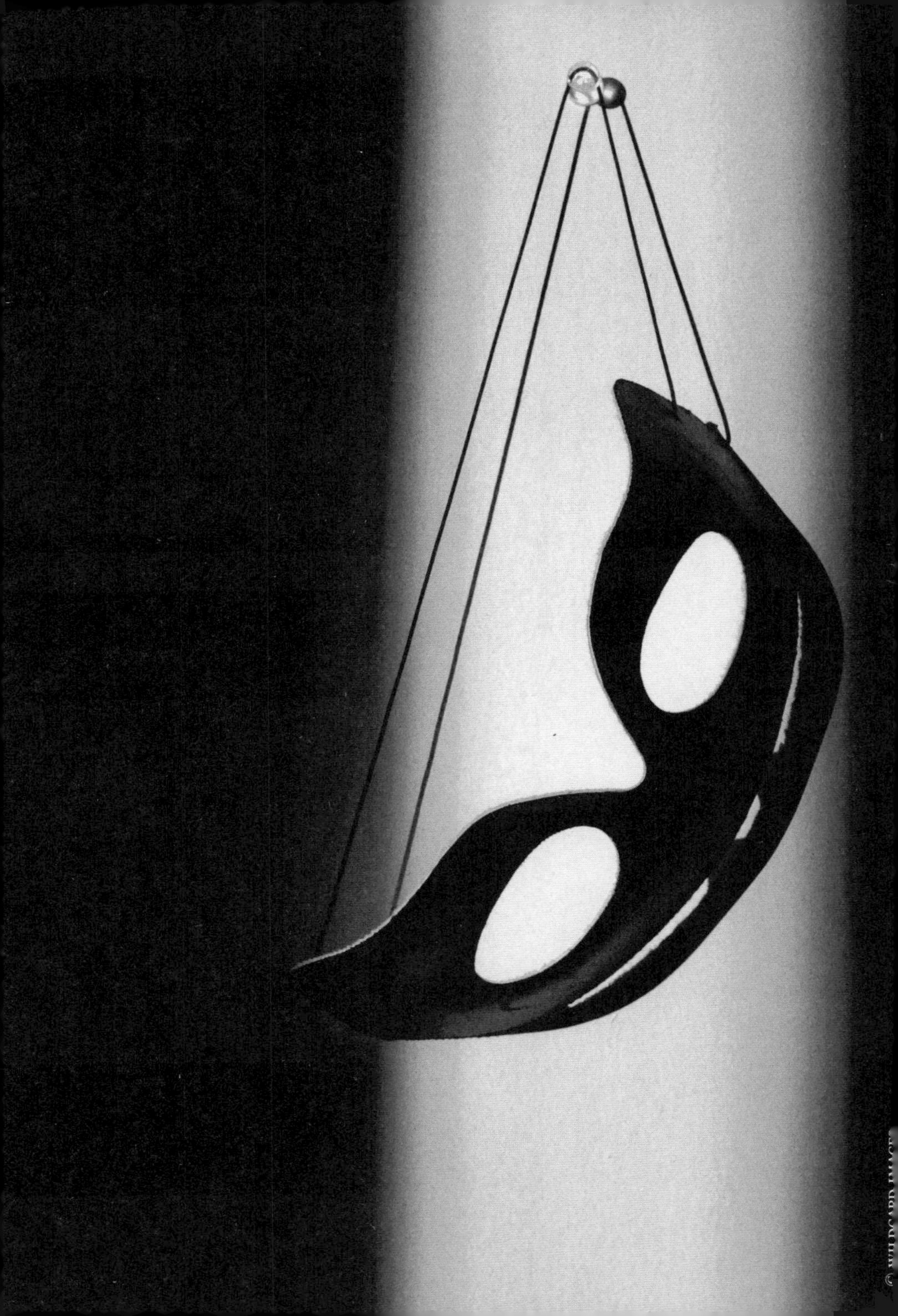

At Gregori's, once you've paid your twenty dollars and checked your clothes and shoes with the friendly men in the antechamber to the left, you are given a mask – the small black kind, like Zorro's. Stretch the elastic a little, you're told, then slip the mask on carefully; there are only enough to go around and they break easily. Once it's on, you hear your own breathing. The almond-shaped openings restrict the field of vision a little: you look straight ahead, the periphery of your gaze softens in an oval of darkness. Now you're ready to enter the party.

Gregori has other parties every Friday night, with a carefully cultivated guest list of men he's met online or in clubs, or guys who've approached him because they've heard about his gatherings. You have to be invited, and the invitation, presumably, is important to the legality of the party – it underscores the fact that this is a private event, held in a private apartment, so this isn't a business subject to regulation, but simply a gathering. Gregori wants at least to see a photo of you or to get a recommendation from someone he knows, but in truth the parties are attended by a wide variety of men: young and lean guys who look like they take yoga classes many times a week, musclemen with their rubbery, steroidal curves, older guys into leather or with a kind of military style, and plenty of men who haven't seen the inside of a gym lately. The men are predominately white or Latin, a few Asians; the only black guy around is one of Gregori's beautiful helpers, a six-foot chiselled tower in red briefs who mans – there could be no other verb! – the door.

But the masked party happens once a month only. The masks don't hide much; were there an acquaintance or a co-worker behind one, you wouldn't have trouble recognizing him. But sometimes a gesture in the direction of anonymity is all that's required. Gregori says the party draws married and bisexual men, actors, guys on the down-low, who feel, between the dim lighting and the slight veil, free. They pose or rest or couple in the soft light washing down from a video screen hung high up on the walls of the two-storey room. (They triple, I want to say, or otherwise multiply, but I need to wash 'couple' and 'multiply' free of the weight of their heterosexual imagery. Little is limited here to two, and nothing will be conceived but possibility.) The men clothed only in the black fabric framing their eyes look strangely Venetian, as though Tiepolo had made secret frescoes of an eighteenth-century sex party.

How has Gregori found these men? A bisexual pal of his goes to clubs in Manhattan patronized by swinging straight couples, and when one of the guys is clearly attracted to him, he gives him Gregori's card. Gregori cruises online sites to find the guys who'd be pleased by the prospect of a veil. If the masks, in a few hours, are worn loosely around the neck like collars, or strewn on the floor beside the sofa, left on a tabletop – well, their work is done. They have opened the doors of the evening, have announced an intent, and now they are no longer necessary.

I dream, as I'm setting out to write this, that I'm walking in a weedy and tangled area in the back of my garden, a part I've never really attended to much, when I discover that there's a neglected path that goes on, opening out further than I knew, and there are daffodils already sprouting, though it's still late in the winter, and the rough beds lead right down to the bay. I didn't know we bordered open water! But I can go further, up an easy slope out of the garden, where you can see across a valley where sheep are sporting and then the path runs on behind the field to a town I think I recognize, but once I'm there I realize it's a town I've never seen. It's clear that home is so much larger and more unfamiliar than I knew.

I have been a masked man – not for a long time now, but there was a period in my life, in my twenties, when I – how to say it? – lived in hiding, lived a double life, was sexually duplicitous? All problematic terms. I was married to a woman and having sex with a man. I imagine that I would have been terrified of Gregori's party, had there been such a thing in Des Moines; I can't imagine myself then being able to move to that level of unselfconsciousness, that degree of abandon. Would that even have been what I wanted? I imagined that one man, one incendiary, generous, open-spirited man, would entrance me, one broad chest would give me a place to lay my head. And, for a time, he did.

Then why on earth was I married?

When I was seventeen, a freshman in college living in my parents' house, I met Ruth at a poetry reading. She was short, blonde, her body rounded like her vowels, her voice forged in central Louisiana and revised in Houston. In some anonymous lounge in the student centre she was part of a reading by a group of grad students; her poems were imagistic, fragmented, and to my ear compellingly weird, as if they emerged from some interior cave still wet with the stuff of dream life. I liked Blake and García Lorca, André Breton and Charles Simic, so of course I liked her, and I went up after to tell her so, and she exclaimed, *Mark, I'm so glad to see you!*, though we'd never met, and I took that as a sign.

A week later I saw her again, at a party at my poetry professor's beautiful house in the desert. We got drunk on Scotch, talked for hours in a state of increasing enrapturement, and made out in my car. 'Made out' is deceptively casual. I think it must have felt momentous to me: I must have felt I was doing something I was supposed to do. These statements are speculative because I feel, in some sense, I wasn't there: I was giving myself up to a current, I wasn't making a decision, I was being carried in the direction the world intended – did I think then it was the world that meant this life for me? She said, 'I feel like an Easter egg.' I loved that. I was seventeen, and to be touched or kissed by anyone was thrilling. I'd had sex exactly twice, in the men's room in the basement of the Liberal Arts building. My art-history class – where we studied slide after slide of classical nudes, and my teacher duly appraised their proportions and poses – was right down the hall, and so I'd go from those perfected marble boys to the intricate graffiti of the stalls, their walls pierced by glory holes, and the hungry mouths and eyes on the other side. You could see just a single eye, or if the man on the other side sat back and you put your eye to the hole, you might see him stroking an erect cock, the startling trembling fact of it, exposed for you there in this public place. I was powerless in the face of my lust, but I was terrified too. Was this the life opening in front of me? My father had warned me about queers, to be wary of men who asked me to go home with them, and that was as much of a conversation as we'd had on the subject. My mother had given vent to her disgust at homosexual intercourse (though it couldn't really be distinguished from the rage and distaste she seemed to feel for the heterosexual variety, too).

In a month or two I told Ruth I was bisexual, which I may have believed. I was, in fact, 'bisexual', since I was having sex with her and thinking about men, but I don't think that's quite what the term is meant to connote. She seemed to experience this information as something absurd, and told me I was mistaken, and then we didn't talk about it again for years. We were living together by summer, and one day she said, rather petulantly, *My friends all want to know when we're going to get married.* I said, *October*? And that was that. There were maybe thirty guests in our apartment, at the wedding – including my parents and our poetry teacher – and we had champagne and cake on the terrace, popping the corks toward Arizona Mortuary across the street and watching as the bats flew out from the roof at twilight.

Judith Butler says heterosexuality is an inevitable comedy because no one can really fulfil the absurd expectations for the categories defined as 'man' and 'woman'. Perhaps more accurate to say that all sexuality is a comedy, since we are bound to codes that forever fail to describe quite who we are, no matter what, and though these externals constitute a portion of our subjectivity (how can I not, to some degree, be the gay man I'm told I am?), they're never entire, thank goodness, never circumscribe us entirely.

It was clear from the beginning that my marriage would be a painful comedy. I drove Ruth to school one day to her afternoon class and pulled into a gated parking lot so I could take her right up to the steps of the building, and before I could even ask, the attendant said, *Oh, do you just want to drop your mother off?* I hadn't understood that's how we'd be seen. One night I came home late from some place or another, and there was a guy hanging out under a street light in front of a bar down the block, a place called the Graduate. I knew it was a gay bar, but just seeing this boy – a hundred yards away perhaps – nobody would have had to tell me: even this far away his school-letter jacket was glowing with desire; he was facing in my direction, we were sending some beam to one another entirely undetectable by any means other than the human body, his white-sleeved jacket a sweet hungry icon. I turned and went into the house. I was eighteen and alive with longing, and I turned and went into the house and lay down beside my sleeping wife.

Which makes me want to say now that I was a stupid boy. Smart when it came to reading, to talking about books and films and especially poems, those spells and chants and passageways into the underlife I loved, but about how to live or how to honour my own heart or my own loins I knew nothing at all.

The comedy deepened. Ruth told me she had a son, by her previous marriage, of whom she'd lost custody, and that this was the great loss of her life. Where was he? I wanted to know. Living with his grandparents now, in Arkansas. She waited until we were married to tell me she had a son? Because we were moving to Iowa, where she'd gotten a teaching job, we could stop along the way, and I could meet him, which meant that she had to tell me how old he was. I was eighteen, and so was my stepson.

You will perhaps see why a writer who has had a good deal to say about other periods of his life has considered this material unwriteable: it seems Gothic, ridiculous. To narrate those years seems inevitably to accuse Ruth, and to invite me to offer justifications for my own foolishness in marrying her. We did what we did. It amazes me, it makes me think of Milosz's unforgettable line about the weight of history: 'I ask not in sorrow but in wonder.' It is indeed wonder that I feel, that this absurd life took place, and yet it's true that I can't return to it without a certain degree of rage, too, and a memory of that ferocious, self-enclosed longing. There was a clock, downtown, on the top of a skyscraper, that flashed its numbers all night long; you could see it from the bedroom of our apartment. 1.27, 1.33... How many nights did I watch those numbers, during the hours when there were only three of them?

Why write this now? Because Alex is dead, just this week, of cancer. My wife is years gone, and now him, and thus of the three of us I live to tell the untold tale, what I promised, at least tacitly, I wouldn't say. Does it need telling? And Alex's wife, maybe she has a story too?

But I get ahead of myself. I met my stepson, on his grandparents' farm in the Arkansas backcountry. He was exactly the boy I was not: six feet two like me, but while I'd been reading Kenneth Patchen and smoking dope, he'd been playing football and digging potatoes. We played like two big dogs who've just met: we swam in the Arkansas, in our cut-off jeans; we wrestled and chased after one another on the bank. With him I was the boy I'd never been, and if what passed between us had nothing of sex in it, it was surely suffused with Eros: all body, and entirely apart from his mother. Then Ruth and I drove to Des Moines, where another life commenced.

The elements of this new existence seemed barely to touch one another at all: I worked in a day-care centre, and became passionately interested in the education of young children; I wrote poetry, at night and on weekends; in the late hours, privately, I burned for the company of men; I attended English Department functions with my wife. It was at one of these, in the impeccably comfortable apartment of a senior English professor of considerable authority named Dr Maurice La Belle, that I met a hairdresser from Iowa City – handsome, ten years older than me, sporting the unmistakable new gay look of the day: tightly curled short hair, a dark moustache, a tan, a lean and well-managed form in tightish clothes. We walked on to a terrace together. He kissed me on the mouth. I was instantly erect – he felt my crotch and pushed his tongue further into my mouth – but I pulled back and said, *For God's sake, my wife is in the next room*. He insisted on giving me his phone number – well, I guess he didn't exactly have to talk me into accepting it. He had no card, and I had nothing handy to write it on, so he inscribed it neatly on the back of my social security card. Which means I have it still, thirty-five years later. Oh, Jim from Iowa City, what are the chances you're still alive, or still at that number?

I was both fleeing from a door that was tumbling open in front of me and, in my less-than-direct way, trying to tug the door open myself. I developed a series of crushes on men who were almost but not quite available: Richard, Hans, guys with a certain vibe of openness or ambiguity who'd become my friends and turn out to be attracted only to women, though they might flirt with me or allow an embrace, even a dry kiss. I'd be spun into dizziness by this, somehow, I thought, satisfied. I had leaned my weight against the door, it hadn't opened, but I could feel some fresh and bracing wind blowing in from the other side.

Then I met the man I'm calling Alex. I need, for reasons which will become clear later on, to becloud some of the circumstances of our encounter. Say we sang in a choir together, lobbied for better funding for social services, sat a few easels away from one another in a drawing class. I remember the pleasure of a long conversation, outdoors, on a cool spring afternoon. We'd started to chat a little, and one joke or story led to another, and soon it became evident, the pleasure we were taking in one another's company. If you'd stood back and watched us, you'd have seen two men in their twenties, both tall, one more lanky and the other a bit thicker, swaying a little as they spoke, hands in their pockets, heads leaning in toward one another, then stepping back to laugh, the conversation going on into the afternoon, one making as though to leave but then stopping again, talking on, the unmistakable physical language of a connection being formed.

We took to going out for beers, playing pinball, listening to bands. This did not fit into the terms of my marriage, where I seemed expected to live like a married man, not like a boy in my early twenties; I think Ruth must have seen my nights out as an annoyance but also a kind of safety valve, or a male zone not unlike my Huck Finn and Tom Sawyer wrestling with her son. In between batting the beautiful chrome balls around their playing fields beneath the glass, we were talking and talking about common acquaintances, politics, work, drawing closer. Then Alex went somewhere or other, on a longish trip, and came back with slides, and to see them I went to his house one evening, a little rented place on the other side of town.

The best place to view the slides was the bedroom; there was a largish bare wall for a screen, and we could put the carousel projector on the bed, and sprawl out on either side of it with a beer while he narrated the images of his journey, and as the pictures progressed our arms and shoulders came closer to one another, and I could feel my own heartbeat, and I was aware, beneath the worn cotton of the tie-dyed T-shirt he wore, of his.

All my life I have looked and looked at the mystery of desire and I feel no closer to understanding it. Nothing else has so shaped my decisions, my way of life; were one to inventory the costs of sexual difference the total would be enormous, yet I know that I would have paid any price. But what is it that compels us, what is it we want? Touch? Entrance behind the barrier of the skin, to penetrate the boundaries of another body, or be penetrated ourselves, as a remedy for our extreme loneliness, the awful sensation of the singular self in the singular skin? Some narcotic form of forgetfulness, an opiate dispensed by the hands of another? Not orgasm, finally, and only partly pleasure: there are many sorts of pleasure, many forms of satisfaction, but what other has the deep lodestone pull that sex has? And I don't believe it's simply biology, the imperative to reproduce – since for me, obviously, there will be no issue from the unions I can't seem to live without. I want; that is the prima facie thing, the ground of being. But what is it, in a man's body, in the heat and touch and warm interior, the rush and delay of contact, what is it that I want? Shouldn't I be able, after a life's worth of practice, to name that?

Here's Whitman, in 'Song of Myself':

Blind loving wrestling touch, sheath'd hooded sharp-tooth'd touch!
Did it make you ache so, leaving me?

Parting track'd by arriving, perpetual payment of perpetual loan,
Rich showering rain, and recompense richer afterward.

But what is the 'recompense richer'? I know that it exists, and I know it resides outside of language, and I know it is not to be denied. We refuse what is originary in ourselves to our peril; what wells up is to be attended to. Blake says, *It is better to murder an infant in its cradle than to nurse desires unacted upon.* This sounds horrifying until you realize that the infant you're killing, if you do not allow your desire to emerge into the daylight, is yourself, the person you might become if you move in the direction of fulfilment. (Not *to* fulfilment, mind you; I no longer believe in that, except as a temporary state, but we need to proceed in satisfaction's direction.)

I was twenty-one years old, and now my real life had started, though I wouldn't have said it that way then. The next morning I was in the bathroom at home, getting ready for work, and Ruth pointed out to me that I was certainly in a good mood, because I was singing. And it was true; I wanted nothing more than to open my mouth and sing.

Once or twice a week, Alex and I would meet, at his place, for sex. In a while he moved to an old apartment building in a neighbourhood nearer to mine, the kind with a rattly cage elevator that cast complicated shadows down the hall, and that's where I always remember him: the candlelit bedroom, a long horizontal mirror beside the bed he kept curtained until it was needed, a bottle of lotion warming in a tub of hot water, music he liked. His song for me was Phoebe Snow, 'Poetry Man', and that kind of jazz-inflected R & B, or the energetic but plaintive Emmylou Harris, that's the sort of soundtrack to those nights. Ardent, inquisitive, exploratory nights. I was the first man he'd had sex with; my own sexual encounters with men before him were merely functional; we had no actual knowledge, and there was joy in creating some. How is it that you could take a long cock into your mouth without gagging, and what were the motions of lips or tongue that would create pleasure? And fucking, that wild taboo mystery of penetration? Alex went first, and almost immediately found that discomfort gave way to radical pleasure. I thought I'd never be able to take anything up my ass; I imagined I just wasn't built that way. But Alex said, *Oh no, if I'm going to do this, you're doing it, too.* And after the initial panic and tension – oh, stars! That same kind of involuntary intake of breath when suddenly you see winter stars spread across a black sky in the country – that scale, that sharp air of possibility.

How can these things ever be inscribed, do they forever belong to the realm of the unwriteable? I have the language of pornography, I have the language of anatomy or medicine, I have the language of euphemism, and I'm happy with none of them.

In Nick Flynn's memoir *Another Bullshit Night in Suck City* there's a list, maybe two or three hundred terms, for being drunk. I could make a list like that for fucking and come absolutely no closer to what I want to say; it is as if the transformative bodily experience lives on one side of the veil and language on the other. What can I say? I fucked him, he fucked me, and then we'd go out and get something to eat and then we'd go back and pick up where we left off. Wild nights, wild nights! – pressurized to diamond-light by secrecy for nearly three years. We never spoke of them to anyone, not a single word.

When I described Gregori's party, I focused on the experience of the man wearing the mask, the one looking out through those restricting apertures. But something happens, too, to the one who is *looking* at the man in the mask. Anything veiled is granted the mysterious capacity to hold more than the uncovered; that which we cannot entirely see becomes the repository of the inarticulate need of the viewer, of inchoate desire. In his book *Stealing the Mona Lisa*, Darian Leader describes how that now-exhausted image became iconic, a pinnacle of Western painting, only after it was stolen from the Louvre, early in the twentieth century; people used to come to view the absence of the picture, gazing into the space where it had hung.

There was a way in which Alex and I partook of this dynamic. I was not, at this point, ready to leave Ruth: a complex web of guilt and shame and misplaced loyalties held me, and Alex shook his head in disbelief at the whole thing but also accepted the situation. And in fact, he did not want to set up housekeeping together: he liked women, too, and began a new relationship while we were still burning up the hours together in our hidden week-night encampments. He said that he couldn't live a gay life, didn't want that stigma; he was from a little Dakota town, and he'd been a freak there all his life, and he'd had judgement enough. How could I judge that, I who'd been wearing my married-man mask for years?

But how open our bodies were to one another! This combination of utter availability and of closed doors – what was his life like when

I wasn't around, or mine without him? – was incendiary; it fuelled our passion, it allowed us to love and to want and to need everything we believed might lie behind the mask.

And it meant, too, that when circumstances changed, so did we. My marriage finally foundered. Ruth's drinking escalated; I'd cover her classes when she was too sick to go, haul the empty bottles back to the state liquor store with increasing horror at their number, watch as she made out with a student on the couch at a party whose theme was the work of Alain Robbe-Grillet. Each guest had been told to arrive at a certain hour – 8.16, 9.27 – and to dress the part, so Ruth and I had gone in formal wear and small black masks, and I'd carried in one hand a toy silver revolver. I pushed us into therapy; I talked and talked – though never about Alex and our affair, not once – until I could name more of what held me in that house where she raged and wept and passed out nightly. We split apart in a firestorm of rage and recrimination; I went to Africa for a month, she to the psych ward, and when I came back I told her it was over and found a cheap little apartment a few blocks away, closer to the university – a dim little place where I cried mightily, and soon found I very much liked living in.

But Alex? We saw each other a few more times, but it was clear all the terms had shifted. I was too available; he was too interested in the woman he was seeing, everything felt wrong, though I liked him as much as I always had and there was this sweet, seemingly permanent thread of friendship stitching us together.

Once, before I was a newly free man, Alex had an accident, on his motor scooter. Nothing was broken but he was bruised and scraped, the skin of his arms and legs and torso battered and scabbed with surface wounds. I went to visit him. He was recovering at a relative's place – though we were alone that afternoon – and he was lying in a big lounge chair, probably a little hazed on painkillers, and so happy to see me. He was wearing just a pair of gym shorts, and after we talked for a while, him narrating the tale of the accident with a grave face, eyes growing wider as he told me how he was knocked off, into the gravel, and how he was unconscious for a while, and what he woke to. Then I knelt beside him to kiss him, first his mouth and then each of his dark nipples, and a bit of unbroken skin on his belly. Then we eased his gym shorts down, and I took his heavy cock in my mouth until it was hard, and sucked it till he came. He was so grateful for these ministrations, he rested his hand on my head and cried.

Now I understand that his body – beautiful though no gym body of a later decade, a broad chest with a rich swath of hair, the beard pointing downward as though to point to the symmetry of his body, the warm total embrace of him – was one of the doors through which I entered my actual life.

I left town, moving on for job and adventure and to distance myself, once I was ready, from the wreckage of my marriage. He married; I saw him and the sweet and funny and open-hearted woman he married later on, and though we talked about much in the past, we never talked about our nights together, and to this day I have no idea what she knew or knows. Thus the need to fog the details here a bit.

Those involved would probably guess anyway, but out of respect for her I want to leave the externals vague. There's no one else to protect. Alex died, just this last week; I learned from a mutual friend I hear from now and then. Ruth died a few years ago; how she survived as long as she did is beyond me. She was one of those substance abusers with a constitution of pure tempered metal, though she spent much of her life professing her weakness and need. If the truth be told, she was something of a pit bull, and we arrived, in time, at the uneasy friendship of people who were married twenty or thirty years ago.

Oh my dears. What would you think, if you saw me at Gregori's, where I've taken on a volunteer job, for one evening, in the clothes–check room, just for the sheer pleasure of helping the desiring, beautiful men out of their street identities and into their nakedness and then into their masks? It gives me so much pleasure, to have this odd social role, to set the men at ease, to usher them into the deeper hours of the night. How would you ever understand the places to which I've travelled? ■

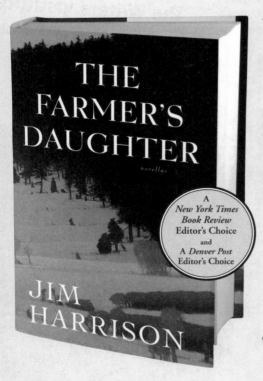

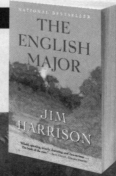

THE REDHEAD

Roberto Bolaño

TRANSLATED BY NATASHA WIMMER

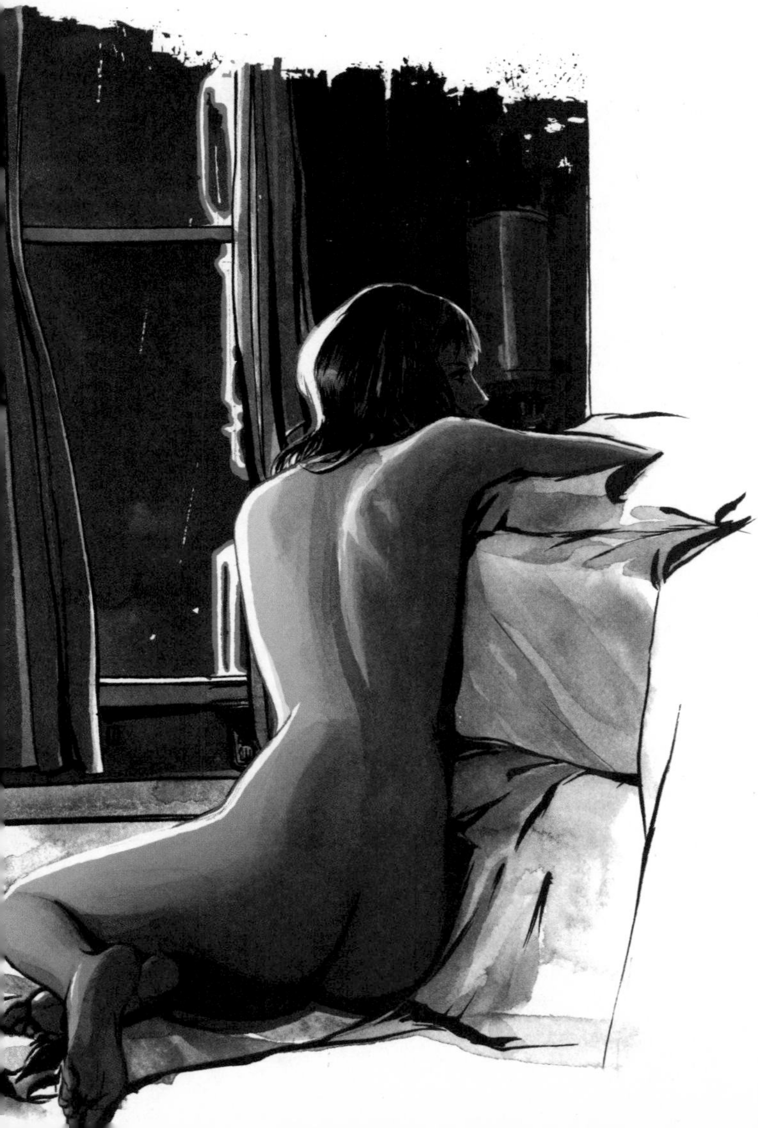

She was eighteen and she was mixed up in the drug trade. Back then I saw her all the time, but if I had to make a police sketch of her now, I don't think I could. I know she had an aquiline nose, and for a few months she was a redhead; I know I heard her laugh once or twice from the window of a restaurant as I was waiting for a taxi or just walking past in the rain. She was eighteen and once every two weeks she went to bed with a cop from the Narcotics Squad. In my dreams she wears jeans and a black sweater and the few times she turns to look at me she laughs a dumb laugh. The cop would get her down on all fours and kneel by the outlet. The vibrator was dead but he'd rigged it to work on electric current. The sun filters through the green of the curtains, she's asleep with her tights around her ankles, face down, her hair covering her face. In the next scene I see her in the bathroom, looking in the mirror, then she says good morning and smiles. She was a sweet girl and she didn't avoid certain obligations: I mean sometimes she might try to cheer you up or loan you money. The cop had a huge dick, at least three inches longer than the dildo, and he hardly ever fucked her with it. I guess that's how he liked it. He stared with teary eyes at his erect cock. She watched him from the bed ... She smoked Camel Lights and maybe at some point she imagined that the furniture in the room and even her lover were empty things that she had to invest with meaning ... Purple-tinted scene: before she pulls down her tights, she tells him about her day... 'Everything is disgustingly still, frozen somewhere in the air.' Hotel-room lamp. A stencilled pattern, dark green. Frayed rug. Girl on all fours who moans as the vibrator enters her cunt. She had long legs and she was eighteen, in those days she was in the drug trade and she was doing all right, she even opened a bank account and bought a motorcycle. It may seem strange but I never wanted to sleep with her. Someone applauds from a dark corner. The policeman would snuggle up beside her and take her hands. Then he would guide them to his crotch and she could spend an hour or two getting him off. That winter she wore a red knee-length wool coat. My voice fades, splinters. She was just a sad girl, I think, lost now among the multitudes. She looked in the mirror and asked, 'Did you do anything nice today?' The cop from Narcotics walked away down an avenue of larches. His eyes were cold, sometimes I saw him in my dreams sitting in the waiting room of a bus station. Loneliness is an aspect of natural human egotism. One day the person you love will say she doesn't love you and you won't understand. It happened to me. I would've liked her to tell me how to endure her absence. She didn't say anything. Only the inventors survive. In my dream, a skinny old bum comes up to the policeman to ask for a light. When the policeman reaches into his pocket for a lighter the bum sticks him with a knife. The cop falls without a sound. (I'm sitting very still in my room in Distrito V; all that moves is my arm to raise a cigarette to my lips.) Now it's her turn to be lost. Adolescent faces stream by in the car's rear-view mirror. A nervous tic. Fissure, half saliva, half coffee, in the bottom lip. The redhead walks her motorcycle away down a tree-lined street … 'Disgustingly still'…'She says to the fog: it's all right, I'm staying with you' … ■

POEM | CARL PHILLIPS

Undo It

Deep from within the changing colours of a life
that itself keeps changing, I know the leaves prove
nothing – though it
                                        does seem otherwise – about
how helplessness is not a luxury, not a hurt by
now worth all the struggling to take back, but
instead what we each, inevitably, stumble
sometimes into,

                                        and sometimes through … As for
that grove-within-a-grove that desire has, so long,
looked like – *falling*, *proof of nothing*, carrion-birds
clouding the slumped boughs of the mountain ash –

I can almost see again: we'll drown anyway – why not
in colour? You're no more to me a mystery, than I to you.

'*A Country in the Moon* is literary travel writing at its best: elegiac, informative and profound. It's probably the best travel book I will read this year'
Jim Blackburn, *Wanderlust* 'Book of the Month'

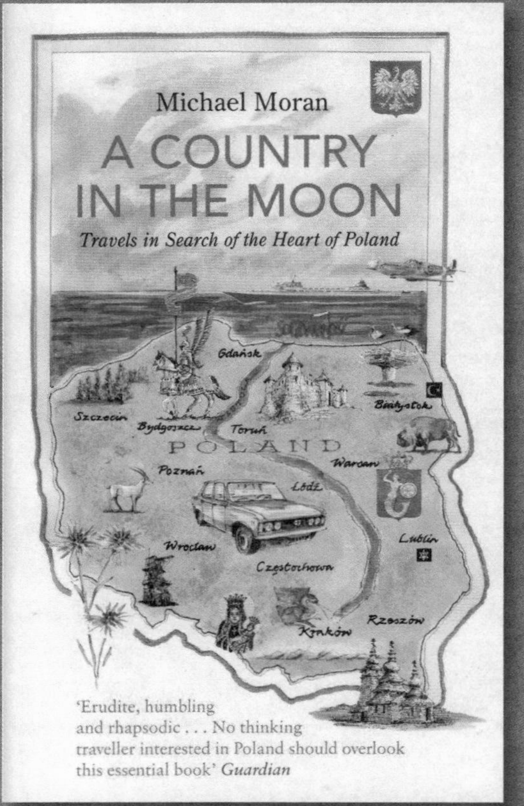

ISBN 9781847081049 • Paperback

'As much cultural history as conventional travel narrative . . . This lively and intelligent book is stuffed with original material that is both fascinating and quite new to most people in the West'
Robert Carver, *Times Literary Supplement*

'Wonderful' Giles Foden, *Condé Nast Traveller*

GRANTA
www.granta.com

GRANTA

TOKYO ISLAND

Natsuo Kirino

TRANSLATED BY PHILIP GABRIEL

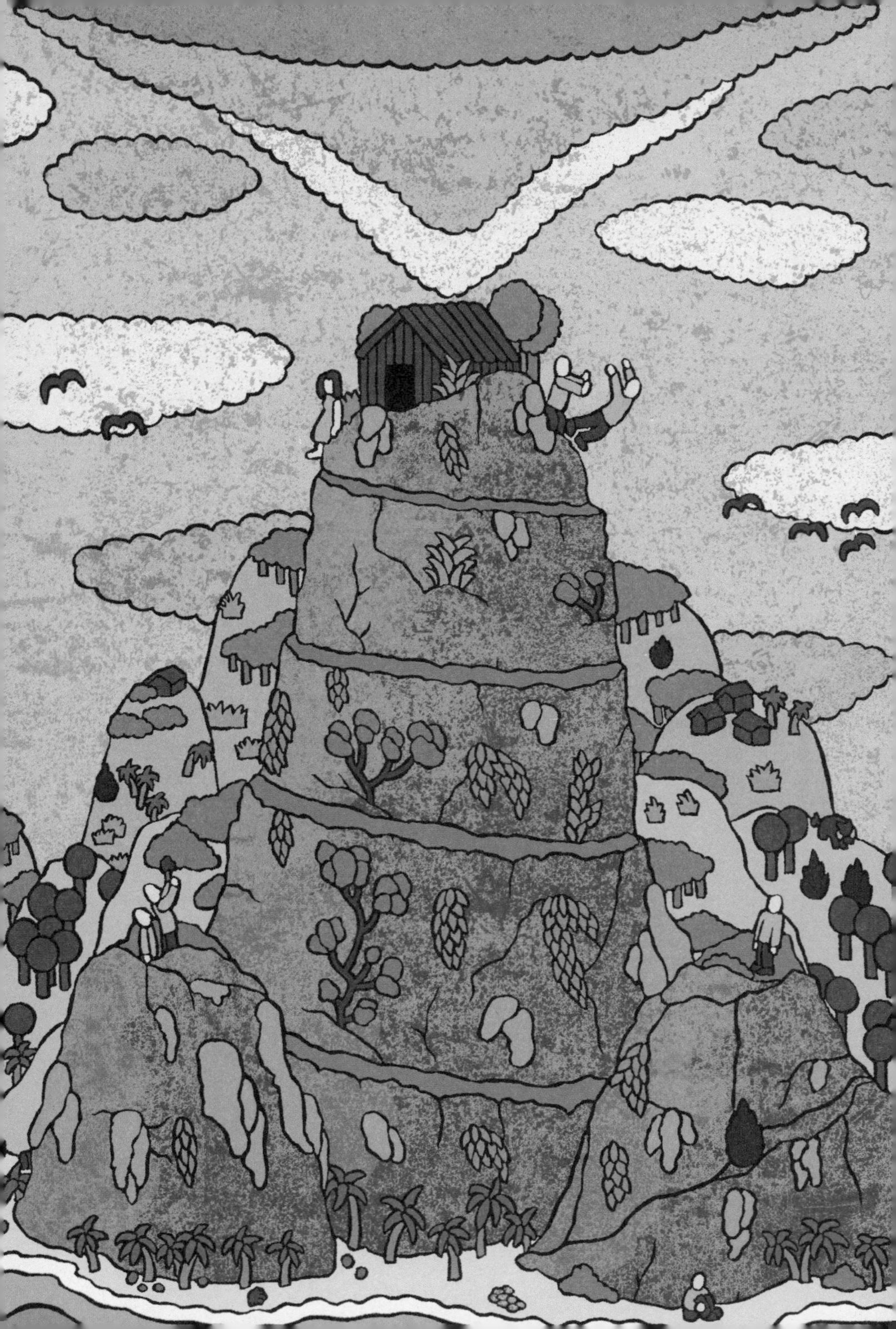

The lottery to choose her next husband was to take place at the Imperial Palace. Kiyoko got up earlier than usual and headed down to Odaiba. The inlet, covered with black stones, was always gloomy, and it was hard to believe it was in the South Seas. Hemmed in by jutting cliffs, the seawater appearing to rise up so much it blocked the entrance, it was an oppressive site. Kiyoko felt locked in and just couldn't bring herself to enjoy the beach. This was the very spot where, five years before, she and her husband Takashi had stumbled ashore after their cruiser had been wrecked. In the midst of a terrible storm, as she spied the island in the distance, she'd been overjoyed, but now she spent each day gazing back out at the ocean knowing she couldn't escape.

Kiyoko removed her tattered black dress and slipped into the sea naked. Swaying in the waves, stepping on the pebbles on the sea floor, she washed her face in the warm water. *I'm the star today so I've got to look my best*, she murmured, an unconscious smile rising to her lips. But Kiyoko was always the star, no matter where she went. People on the island studied her every move, doing their best to stay in her good graces and win her attention, an understandable reaction since among the thirty-two residents of the island she was the only woman. Kiyoko fingered back her tangled hair and tied it with a strand of brown algae. She turned forty-six this year, and though her hair had got a bit thinner, she didn't look her age. In the entire world there must be only a handful of women that men so desperately yearned for.

Three months after she and Takashi had become castaways, twenty-three young Japanese washed up on the island. They were part-time workers, all men, who had been hired to investigate the wild horses living on Yonaguni Island. The work – collecting horse manure, mashing it and looking for parasite eggs – was tiring, dirty and their pay was bad. Unable to stand it any more, they stole a nearly derelict boat and escaped. As luck would have it, though, they ran into a typhoon and were cast adrift, eventually crawling ashore here. Takashi and Kiyoko had stayed up the whole night rescuing these men from the dark sea. They were happy they had new companions, but the young men's arrival only meant there were more people locked away on the island. They still didn't know which country this island belonged to, or what its name was – none of the young men had any idea. And as before, no one came to rescue them.

Somewhere along the line the young men began to call the island Tokyo-jima – Tokyo Island. Takashi made fun of the name, disparaging it as their misplaced nostalgia for home, but Kiyoko saw in it the determination of the young men, if they couldn't go home, to at least create their own version of home – a kind of pseudo-Tokyo – and enjoy themselves. Kiyoko knew exactly how they felt.

Kiyoko gazed back at the island, the low hills covered with thick vegetation. Takashi had surveyed the island and reported that it was seven kilometres long and four kilometres wide, and shaped like a crushed kidney. There weren't any poisonous snakes or bobcats or other dangerous creatures, but plenty of wild bananas, taro potatoes and coconuts. Aside from the fact that it was a deserted island and no one was about to come and rescue them, it was, arguably, a kind of paradise.

Sensing something, Kiyoko turned round and found three Hong Kongers standing there. All three had faint smiles as they stared at her naked body. She recognized them, of course, but didn't know their names. One of them made a beach-ball gesture with his hands to indicate how fat she was. Angered, Kiyoko turned away. Kiyoko was, indeed, the chubbiest person on the island. Why this impoverished life should make her put on the pounds, she had no idea. Her plump body was proof that life on the island agreed with her, and she hated it.

One morning three years back, one of the islanders spotted a ship anchored offshore and they had all raced down to the beach. They yelled at the top of their voices and waved their hands.

Some of them yanked off their T-shirts, tied them to the ends of sticks and waved these makeshift flags madly. Eventually an inflatable yellow boat was lowered from the bow of the ship and the island's residents went wild. Some collapsed in tears; some scooped up pebbles and stuffed them into their pockets as a last memento, while others raced about in every direction, insanely overjoyed. But this boat wasn't there to rescue them. On board was a sailor holding a rifle, and at least ten other people, all with dark hair, depressed and dejected figures, hunched over like criminals. Threatened by the sailor with the rifle, the men were forced to disembark and wade ashore. The now-emptied inflatable boat spun round and headed back to the ship. The islanders stood there, stunned, and soon began to shout hysterically: 'Help us! We're Japanese!' But without giving so much as a glance in their direction, the ship sailed away from the inlet, never to return.

The ten men left on shore were dressed in shorts and running shirts and had no belongings. They stared, disappointedly, at the sobbing Japanese, and then plonked down on the shore, sighing deeply and murmuring among themselves. A few stretched out on the beach.

The guy they called Atama – literally, *head* – a former member of a motorcycle gang, attempted to communicate with the new arrivals, but they didn't understand him. 'Seems like they're Chinese,' the islanders whispered to each other. Atama took a stick and wrote *Chinese*? in the sand in characters, and the new arrivals all nodded. He then wrote *Which island*? and the oldest of the group, a man in his forties, grabbed the stick and wrote three characters in response. Compared to Atama's lousy characters the older man's handwriting was beautiful, but none of the Japanese could decipher it. Later, they learned that the ten men had stowed away on a ship headed to Japan and because of trouble over money had been forcibly abandoned on the island.

With the Chinese group's appearance, the Japanese community became more united, though nothing positive came of it. The Japanese decided that the Chinese must be a pretty disreputable lot to have been abandoned on the island like that, and contempt for them only reinforced their own sense of pride at how they had all survived a storm and managed to make it ashore on their own power. In the end, though, they figured such differences mattered little, for they were all stuck in the same miserable circumstances. Besides, the reality of having to struggle to survive on this deserted island had made the Japanese so lethargic and aloof that a different culture and people was the last thing they cared about. Since the Chinese men's arrival, the western part of the island that the Japanese group lived in (the part with an indented shoreline) had been dubbed Tokyo; the eastern part where the Chinese lived was called Hong Kong. Odaiba was the lower part of the kidney shape and was a joint harbour – a harbour in name only, though, since it was unlikely any more ships would ever show up.

The Hong Kongers quickly adjusted to life on the island, as if they'd been there for years. They were coarse and crude, scattering their garbage everywhere and urinating and defecating with abandon. Since their community was entirely male, they went around naked most of the time and blended into the jungle scenery like a new species of wild animal. But in terms of sheer will to survive, the Tokyoites were no match for them. Both groups prized rats and lizards as valuable sources of protein, but while the Tokyoites would eat them as soon as they snagged them, the Hong Kongers kept these creatures in cages and painstakingly bred them. When they caught small fish, they coated them with seawater and dried them in the sun to preserve them, breaking them into pieces for soup stock and coming up with numerous new recipes. Wonderful smells emanated from Hong Kong village, and a calm, peaceful feeling that belied the reality of life on a deserted island. There was even an epicurean side to them – they had an amazing ability to locate edible ingredients, and it was rumoured that they had found wild garlic and peppers and were using these to spice up their meals.

There was only one thing that Tokyo could boast about to the Hong Kongers: the fact that they had the only woman on the island, albeit a middle-aged one.

Kiyoko was the only one of the Japanese the Hong Kongers seemed to care about, observing her closely, giving her food and trying to entice her to visit their village. For Kiyoko, it mattered little whether they were Hong Kongers or Tokyoites, middle-aged men or inexperienced boys – all the other islanders belonged to the race of males, and she was the only female. They might fight over her, Kiyoko thought, but her very fragility, her status as an endangered species, would keep them from ever harming her. On Tokyo Island she was the equivalent of the *toki*, the Japanese crested ibis, a rare bird on the verge of extinction.

The Hong Kongers removed their filthy shorts and underwear, and carefully buried them in the sand, marking each person's spot with a stone. They did this so the wind wouldn't blow their clothes away. Clothes were the hardest item to keep in supply on the island, and the Hong Kongers stripped naked whenever they worked. Kiyoko stared at the men's penises, to see if viewing her naked body had produced any reaction, but found none. They were totally focused on gathering food, their expressions deadly serious as they exchanged a few last-minute instructions before plunging into the sea. They all grasped harpoons made of sharpened branches. The only fish in this harbour were small, bony and unpalatable, and the Tokyoites had long since given up on them, but the Hong Kongers never ignored a potential source of nourishment.

The Hong Kongers, naked, began to spear fish and Kiyoko got out of the water. As she let her wet body dry in the breeze, she pondered the banquet that evening, what delicacies she would eat and how much fun it would be. There would be steamed bananas, taro dumplings, coconut wine, lizard steaks. Kiyoko started to salivate at the idea. And she began to enjoy imagining who would end up being her husband. It had been a month since her third husband, Noboru, had left.

Kiyoko returned to her shack, built on the highest point of the island, a shack she had named Chofu, after the affluent residential area in Tokyo. The first thing she did was report back to her husband's mortuary tablet. This wasn't a regular Buddhist mortuary tablet, the kind you find in front of family altars, but a simple white stone with his name scraped on it with a burnt piece of wood.

'Takashi, I'm going to get married today. I never imagined I'd get married four times. Please keep watch over me from heaven, OK?'

A little over a year after she and Takashi had washed up on the island, he'd died mysteriously, falling from the cliffs at Cape Sainara (the name a variant of *sayonara*) on to the boulders below. Rumour had it that her second husband, Kasukabe, had been jealous of Takashi and had pushed him off the cliff, but this didn't bother Kiyoko. She much preferred Kasukabe to Takashi. As long as they were on this deserted island, it was only to be expected that people would disappear one by one. Takashi's turn just came early, that's all.

It was five years before, in June, that Takashi and Kiyoko had departed in their cruiser from Naha Harbour in Okinawa on their round-the-world trip. Kiyoko had complained about having to live aboard a boat for a year, and Takashi had made extravagant promises to convince her to come. 'After our adventures in ports of call all over the world,' he explained, 'we'll settle down in Australia.' Anticipating downsizing in his company, Takashi had been offered a 20 per cent extra early-retirement package and had quit his job immediately. He was forty-seven at the time. Kiyoko was left uneasy about living aboard a boat and anxious about the future. She also worried about her own judgement, for she'd never noticed until now how self-centred her husband was. Takashi was experienced with yachts and full of confidence, and he worked her hard while they were on board. Still, life is hard to fathom, for only three days into their voyage they encountered a hellacious storm and drifted for several days. While they drifted, Takashi was courageous, never giving up, and bolstering Kiyoko's flagging spirits. As soon as they reached the island, however, there was a complete role reversal. Kiyoko's survivor instincts came to the fore as she dug up taro roots, tasted plants that looked like Malabar spinach, and caught and skinned snakes, while Takashi, who had a sensitive stomach, suffered from food poisoning and grew gaunt and weak. Eventually he was reduced to drinking coconut wine and lying in bed all day. And as soon as the party of young men came ashore he turned jealous, claiming that Kiyoko was shamelessly flirting with them. *It's a good thing he died before meeting the Hong Kongers*, Kiyoko thought with a gentle smile. He wouldn't have been able to stand it.

Kasukabe was still a young man of twenty-one when she married him. He'd got sick of his job as a plasterer and applied to work at the job in Yonaguni Island, but until the day he died he kept on muttering how he'd rather have his boss beat him than have taken that job. Even with Takashi around he didn't hesitate to hit on Kiyoko, and they made love any number of times. For Kiyoko the relationship was both troubling and joyful. Loving a man young enough to be her own son was a happiness she'd never experienced before, but Kasukabe also had a ferocious, merciless side to him and he detested all the other men who chased after Kiyoko and picked fights with them. Kasukabe died two years ago, in the middle of the night. Like Takashi, he fell to his death at Cape Sainara. It had hurt Kiyoko badly, for she had truly loved him. After Kasukabe's death, Kiyoko completely transformed her self-image. Now she saw herself as an evil woman who drove men to their deaths. She became intoxicated with the feeling of herself as a woman young men would beg for, one whose very existence brings on tragedy. Kasukabe's death changed everything on the island.

Atama and Oraga had come to Kiyoko's house, entreating her to choose her next husband. 'I don't have anybody I particularly like,' she smiled, and after exchanging a glance they said: 'Then let's have a lottery to choose who will be your next husband.' The term for a husband would be two years, they said, and after that there would be another lottery. It sounded like the slave trade to her, but she went along with it. This was after the Hong Kongers had arrived on the island and the Tokyoites' desire to shore up their group solidarity was at its height; Kiyoko wasn't brazen enough to oppose the wishes of the community.

Her third husband, Noboru, was chosen this way, by lottery. Noboru had barely finished junior high school and was the kind of stupid boy whose only skills were squatting outside convenience stores and flashing a meaningless V-sign. On top of which, he was lazy.

Kiyoko felt like she was saddled with a worthless son, and more times than not wanted to kick him out of the house.

Kiyoko said a wordless goodbye to her three husbands and slipped out of her black dress. From the shelf she took down one of Takashi's shirts and a pair of chino shorts. They were yellowed and ripped in places, but were the least damaged of her clothes. She took good care of them, thinking that, if by any miracle they were rescued, this would be the outfit she would wear.

All the residents of Tokyo Island were already assembled in the plaza in front of the Imperial Palace (a simple structure, four pillars covered over with coconut leaves): three from Bukuro, four from Juku, the six from Shibuya, two from Kitasenju, two from Chiba and two others who lived alone. Nineteen in all. Watanabe, the sole resident of Tokaimura, couldn't be reached. A strictly run lottery would take place among those who had applied to determine who would be Kiyoko's next husband. The young men looked solemn as soon as they spied Kiyoko in full dress – or was she only imagining it? Inukichi, decked out in a shell necklace and a series of bracelets made of palm nuts, pointed behind them.

The Hong Kongers had suddenly materialized below the hill on which the Imperial Palace plaza stood. And Watanabe was among them. Kiyoko hadn't seen him in a while, and though his hairline had receded a bit, he seemed to still have all his teeth. Watanabe watched her closely, his usual sneer on his face. He had a running shirt plastered to his skinny frame, the shirt so filthy it was impossible to tell its original colour. His lustreless hair waved in the sea breeze.

Yan, one of the Hong Kongers, dressed in black shorts, raised a hand in greeting and smiled to no one in particular, as if in anticipation of something amusing to come. Strong-looking yellow canines were visible in his mouth. Yan motioned with his chin. The middle-aged man she'd run across in Odaiba that morning reverently brought forward a lump of something wrapped in banana leaves. The fragrance of meat hit them and commotion ran through the Tokyoites. 'Wild boar, it's wild-boar meat!' A whisper ran through the crowd. The middle-aged man wrote in the sandy soil with a stick. *Congratulations*, it read. As always, the handwriting was superb. Oraga, seeing that Atama didn't know the characters, wrote a reply. *Sye sye* – thank you.

Thanks, Atama said, taking the chunk of meat, and the others watched impatiently as he unwrapped it. It looked like a thigh portion, grilled to perfection. Immediately, Kiyoko's senses were drunk on the prospect of having real animal protein for the first time in ages. Not protein from lizards or snakes, but grilled, boneless wild boar. The Tokyoites were shocked at this display of the Hong Kongers' abilities. Even Watanabe looked a bit plumper than in the past.

In a solemn tone, Oraga, the master of ceremonies, spoke.

'We have solicited candidates for the lottery, and I was wondering, Kiyoko, if you'd care to say a few words.'

'No matter what, don't include Watanabe or Noboru,' she replied.

Noboru turned away, while Watanabe chuckled. Oraga pushed up his glasses, which had slipped down, and looked confused. The frames of his glasses had broken long ago and he kept them on with vines wrapped around his head, which made him look particularly odd.

'You heard the lady. Now, everybody who wants to participate in the lottery please raise your hand.'

There was silence for a moment. Kiyoko looked up to see how many there were. One, two, three – six altogether. She was frankly disappointed there were this few. Not counting Chibi and his gay partner, and her former husband Noboru, that left sixteen men. Even Inukichi, whom she'd fellated so often, didn't raise his hand and was gazing out at the ocean. Kiyoko bit her lip in humiliation.

Six clamshells lay on the ground, one for each of the candidates. They would open them one by one, starting in order of age; the one with a mark on the inside would be the new groom. The men who'd raised their hands were in high spirits, as if playing a game, as they opened the shells. The lottery two years before had been a much more solemn, tense affair, Kiyoko recalled in chagrin. The lottery was won by the fourth in line, G. M. He was thought to be twenty-seven or twenty-eight.

When he was working on Yonaguni Island, G. M. claimed he was a student at a provincial public university. Nobody knew, though, if it was the truth, since the shock of washing ashore here had left him with amnesia. The belongings he had with him all had the initials G. M., so that's what they called him. Much later on, Kiyoko heard that when they were on Yonaguni Island he'd been outgoing, a group leader, but she found this hard to believe since on their island he was so taciturn and inconspicuous. He belonged to none of the groups and made his living as a masseur. Kiyoko had had him massage her a number of times, but wasn't too impressed with his skill at finding the pressure points.

'Make us proud, G. M.!'

As the bearded young men congratulated him, G. M. glanced confusedly over at Kiyoko. Only three of the men had never shared Kiyoko's bed, and G. M. was one of them. When they were picking lots, he was the only one who looked like he was taking it seriously, Kiyoko mused. She felt at once expectant and uneasy about having him as her new husband. Would he be good at making love? Would he be enough for her?

'We now turn to the wedding ceremony for Kiyoko and G. M.,' Oraga announced. There was a scattering of applause, and with the abundance of coconut wine on hand the partygoers soon grew festive. The Hong Kongers hesitantly, but steadily, edged forward to the circle of revellers. They'd brought the wild boar, after all, and couldn't be ignored, so Oraga motioned them forward. Yan came first, clapped G. M. on the shoulder and said something to him, no doubt words of congratulation. Next he went to Kiyoko and clapped her on the shoulder. As he did, his fingers, with their grubby fingernails, stealthily crept over her neck. Kiyoko turned and Yan whispered something in her ear. *Come over to Hong Kong and we'll show you a good time*, she imagined. She pictured herself in his arms and suddenly felt hot. Living like this, as the only woman on the island, had transformed her into a simmering cauldron of desire far greater than the sum of all the men around her, a desire that could swallow the entire island and still not be fulfilled.

'Kiyoko,' Watanabe said to her. 'Come on over to Hong Kong. It's much more fun than being with this lot.'

'What's so fun about it?'

'All sorts of things. I can't tell you here. But they're working on an amazing project.'

Watanabe didn't elaborate and shot a glance at the Hong Kongers behind them. *Are they raising wild boar?* Kiyoko wondered. Or maybe they've designed traps to catch bats? Catching bats was next to impossible.

'What is it? Tell me,' she insisted.

'I will if you let me do you.'

'Are you kidding? I just got married, for God's sake.'

'You can talk,' Watanabe sneered. 'You're the slut of the island. You're an old bag, your privates all slack and flabby, but since you're the only woman around everybody falls all over you.'

Kiyoko felt her blood rise, but it wouldn't help getting angry at this person everyone hated, so she laughed it off.

'Go ahead and laugh, you idiot. Just try and make a fool of me!'

Watanabe grumbled a parting shot and went to sit down with the Hong Kongers. If Watanabe were the last man left, Kiyoko decided, that would be the end of sex on the island.

Halfway through the banquet, the new couple was to leave and head to Kiyoko's house to spend their first night together. Yan raised his hand and said something. Watanabe proudly interpreted.

'He says that at the next lottery in two years he'd like you to let the Hong Kongers participate. We have a right to, he says, because we're contributing to the development of the island.'

Oraga, his eyes red from the coconut wine, asked Kiyoko. 'What do you think, Kiyoko?'

The Tokyoites, taken aback, looked to Kiyoko for her reaction. If she consented, the Tokyoites wouldn't like it, but turning the Hong Kongers down would hurt their feelings. It was a real dilemma.

'How do you feel about it?' Kiyoko countered.

'We can't say anything – it's entirely up to you.'

Ever since she'd married her third husband, none of this was up to her any more, she felt, but here she was being asked to decide about the Hong Kongers' proposal. The Tokyoites' cunning depressed her.

'I'll have to think about it,' she smiled, her expression showing she was deliberately putting them off, and Watanabe translated. Yan glared at Kiyoko with his piercing eyes. She felt terrified, worried what the malicious Watanabe might have told him.

The sun had set and the road to Chofu was dark. When she looked back she saw the red bonfire in the Imperial Palace plaza. Shadowy figures were dancing around it, yelling out. Kiyoko felt exhausted. The only woman on the island also happened to be the oldest person on the island. Her new husband, G. M., followed her without a word.

'Don't you ever talk?' she asked.

She took him by the hand and felt it trembling. *What's the matter?* she wondered. *This isn't a human sacrifice or anything.* Kiyoko was angry. These young men were just using her. They used her when they wanted to, but employed this method designed to downplay any fights over her, and to hold Kiyoko's wildness in check. The Tokyoites had pushed Kasukabe off the cliff, she was sure of it, but where was that knowledge going to get her? The happiness she'd been feeling was quickly deserting her, and Kiyoko sadly made her way into her hut. It was dim inside, but too much trouble to light a fire, so she plopped down on her newly made bed stuffed with dry coconut leaves. With all the wine she'd drunk, her legs felt wobbly.

'I'm exhausted. You know, I can never figure out what you men are thinking. Do you actually need me any more, or am I just superfluous?'

G. M. didn't reply. Time passed and Kiyoko fell asleep. In the middle of the night she suddenly found it hard to breathe and woke up. G. M. was on top of her, clinging to her breasts. 'So it's begun,' she said, as gently as she could.

'You're heavy. Don't just jump right in, OK?'

But G. M. still clung to her, trembling. He was crying. Kiyoko, startled, looked at his face in the moonlight. His scraggly beard formed a dark shadow. G. M. wiped away his tears and said, 'I'm sorry. I just felt so lonely all of a sudden. This is the first time I've slept with anybody since I came to the island, and I finally understand.'

'Understand what?'

'How horribly lonely I've been.'

'Everybody's lonely.'

'It's not that simple. You don't understand …'

G. M. curled up like a baby and snuggled against her. The narrow bed creaked. Not that it was poorly made – Sakai, the former carpenter's apprentice, had constructed it out of interlocking boards, and it was the sturdiest, most luxurious bed on the island. Sakai had an ulterior motive in doing this favour, of course, hoping to use the bed himself with Kiyoko.

'Really? As the only woman here I've been pretty lonely myself.'

'When I managed to swim ashore here,' G. M. said, 'I was so relieved I just lay on the beach and couldn't move. *I'm saved*, I thought. I slept for a while and after I woke up I had no idea who I was or where I came from. I could speak and knew how to do things; it's just that any memory related to myself was missing. I couldn't remember any of it – my name, my parents, what I did, where I lived. It's terrifying. I can't even remember if I'm Japanese, or who my friends were. All I have are the initials G. M. And it hurts. The only memories I have are ones from this island.'

'You still don't remember anything?'

G. M. nodded. Kiyoko suddenly felt sorry for him and stroked his bony back. He let out a deep sigh.

'Thank you. I'm really sorry.'

'It's OK. You're my husband now. We're family.'

'You don't know how happy that makes me.'

Relieved now, perhaps, G. M. soon began snoring peacefully. At a loss, Kiyoko got out of bed and gazed up through cracks in the palm-thatched roof to the brightly shining moon. She recalled how, two years after they'd come to the island, the men had gone crazy fighting over her. It wasn't just sex they were after. These young men were dying of loneliness. Now that they had found other reasons to live and had come to terms with their loneliness, what would become of her? And how was she supposed to combat her own loneliness? A lottery to pick a husband for her wasn't going to do it. Kiyoko felt like she was going to collapse back on to the bed. She was struck by a terror that shook her to the core: unless she found her own reason for living – something other than sex – she might not survive on this island. She listened to G. M.'s snores. He'd taken over the whole bed now, his body sprawled out, totally at peace. As she watched his sleeping face, she felt a new surge of energy. *I'll help you get your memory back,* she declared. And at this moment she discovered a new purpose in life.

The next morning she sensed someone beside her and woke up. G. M. was standing next to her with a kind of tray he'd fashioned, heaped high with grilled green bananas. He looked sheepish as he watched her wake up.

'Would you like some breakfast?'

How considerate, Kiyoko thought as she got up. *I wish Noboru could see someone working this hard.* G. M.'s face was shining, like she'd never seen it before. He's pretty handsome after all, Kiyoko thought, gazing at him. Unlike the rest of the plain-looking bunch of men on the island, G. M.'s shaved face was striking.

'I feel like I used to do this in the past, and it makes me feel sort of nostalgic.'

'Was there an old person in your house?' Kiyoko hurt herself with the remark. The reality of living with a man twenty years younger than her suddenly oppressed her.

'I'm not sure. I just have a faint memory of taking care of someone.'

'Do you have any idea what the initials G.M. stand for?' Kiyoko asked.

'Who knows?' G. M. said unhappily, inclining his head.

'How about getting a new name? I could give you one.' Kiyoko was surprised by her own suggestion. G. M. looked pleased with the idea. 'How about Yutaka? You look a little like Yutaka Takenouchi, the actor.'

G. M. didn't seem to know who this was, but still he sighed, apparently relieved.

'I feel reborn,' he said. 'And I think I can live on this island now.'

That night Kiyoko and Yutaka consummated their marriage. Making love with him wasn't as intense as with Kasukabe, or as one-sided as with Noboru. Instead it was gentle, sweet and loving. Now that she had Yutaka as a husband, Kiyoko was determined to foster the one thing most missing from the island – namely, love. The problem was that in two years there would be another lottery. Yutaka swore he would protest it, but she didn't seem very confident that he'd prevail. When the other men saw the complete transformation in Yutaka, there would be even more who would clamour to marry Kiyoko so she could make them happy, and the proposal by the Hong Kongers weighed heavily on her. If she turned them down, it might lead to unimaginable troubles.

Married life with Yutaka went almost too smoothly. He was good at getting her to baby him, and on days when Kiyoko wasn't feeling very upbeat he'd sit there, sadly hanging his head until she spoke to him. Kiyoko, completely smitten with him now, would eventually apologize, dipping her chin coquettishly, and Yutaka would relax and smile. Kiyoko was as transformed as he was, and could see her earlier husbands now for what they really were. Putting the idiotic Noboru aside as an exception, she now saw Takashi as a haughty, overconfident banker, and Kasukabe as a mere sex machine. Compared to them, Yutaka was unassuming and gentle, the ideal husband.

One day, three months later, Kiyoko woke up early and headed off for Tokaimura. Tokaimura got its name from the town in Japan that was the site of a huge radiation spill, Japan's own version of Chernobyl. The beach at Tokaimura was littered with dozens of mysterious metal drums, made of a frosted metal like aluminium, with tight yellow lids. Some of the more curious islanders had tried to prise off the lids, but after someone else had wondered aloud if they contained radioactive waste, people were too afraid to approach them. Ever since, they called the beach Tokaimura. Unlike Odaiba, Tokaimura was a beautiful, white-sand beach stretching out as far as the eye could see, and they regretted having to abandon it. But if it was radioactive, avoiding it was the only smart move. The Tokyoites no longer went there, but the white beaches with the shallow waters were ideal for collecting shellfish. Everyone flinched at the thought of getting food from there, fearing it would be radioactive, but the supply of coconuts and bananas was dwindling and unless they went over to the Hong Kong side of the island they wouldn't have enough to eat. She strode through the jungle for some three hours, searching for edible insects and plants as she went, and it was clear to her that compared to a few years before, the supply of food on the island had significantly decreased. It must be because of the Hong Kongers coming here, Kiyoko thought angrily, conveniently overlooking how the Tokyoites had themselves exploited the island's resources.

The beach came into view. But where were all the metal drums? Kiyoko went pale. Could a ship have come without anybody noticing and collected all the drums? *No way*! Her heart was pounding. The Hong Kongers always kept a diligent watch over Tokaimura. A ship could have come and taken all of them away without them ever telling the Tokyoites. Outraged, she felt woozy for a moment, but then she remembered seeing the Hong Kongers at Odaiba that morning. She raced down to the beach and found a lone man there, at the shoreline, staring out to sea.

'Kiyoko, what a surprise.'

It was Watanabe. They hadn't seen him since the wedding ceremony. Watanabe was chewing something, a vacant look in his eyes. The inside of his mouth was red.

'What are you eating?'

'Betel nut.'

'Where did you find it? Tell me.'

Watanabe didn't reply, and smiled as he chomped noisily on the nut. There was a rumour that the Hong Kongers were cultivating tobacco.

The economic disparity between Hong Kong and Tokyo was steadily growing, but if there were any wild betel palms, this was a joint resource. She had to get some, so she asked again.

'Won't you tell me where it's growing? If you do …'

'… You'll let me do you? No thanks. I can get along fine without your snatch.'

What was going on? With a sense of foreboding, Kiyoko trotted down the beach. There were drag marks on the sand where the metal drums had been. The Hong Kongers must have taken them somewhere. She looked around her and spied Yan in the lee of the rocks. He was holding his arms wide apart, in a welcoming gesture, smiling, his yellow teeth showing. Kiyoko nodded to him. What could these guys be up to? Curiosity won out over her apprehension, and she approached him. Yan said something and took her by the hand.

'What are you doing?' she asked. 'And where do you think you're taking me? Remember – I have a husband.'

Watanabe followed after them, snickering. He too tugged Kiyoko by the hand and pointed at something in the lee of the rocks. Kiyoko shouted out loud and fell to her knees in the sand. There were two boats. Next to them lay a fine-looking axe and saw. The Hong Kongers had had nothing, but from the metal of the drum lids they'd fashioned, not weapons, but more useful objects. They'd cut down trees, planed them and constructed these boats. *Well done*! Kiyoko thought, looking at Yan. He said something to her and Watanabe interpreted.

'We're going to escape in these today. You can come with us.'

Astonished, Kiyoko stared at the boats. Watanabe urged her to reply. Yan gazed into Kiyoko's face. His eyes looked cunning, and raunchy. Kiyoko was torn, worried by the thought that she might end up a mere plaything while they were at sea who would be kicked overboard once they tired of her. And besides, she couldn't imagine living apart from Yutaka – that's how happy her fourth marriage had made her. Yan pointed to the jungle behind them and shouted.

'He says that if you stay on the island you'll starve to death. He'll take you because you're a woman, but he won't let any of the other Tokyoites go with them. I think you'd better make a decision pretty quick.'

Watanabe glared at her spitefully. *God, what should I do*? Kiyoko agonized. *Is this a chance to be saved, or will it only end in death?* Her head bowed, Kiyoko struggled to come to a decision. Meanwhile, the Hong Kongers were loading oars and food into the boats. They looked like they were enjoying the work, and she decided that she wouldn't die if she went along with them. If they were rescued, she could get help for those she left behind. If she saw Yutaka again she could explain why it happened. She could always tell him the Hong Kongers had kidnapped her.

Kiyoko raised her head. 'Take me with you.'

Yan gave a satisfied nod and led her by the hand to the bow of one of the boats. Kiyoko grabbed on to the edge and looked up at Tokyo Island. Maybe she was imagining it, but the thick greenery suddenly struck her as shabby. This was most definitely an island on the decline. Bye-bye, everybody. Bye-bye, Yutaka ... Suddenly she remembered the clean shirt and shorts she'd been saving for when she was rescued, and regretted that all she had on was her usual dress. ■

ROUSSEAU AND THE PUSSYCAT

Marie Darrieussecq

TRANSLATED BY EMMELENE LANDON

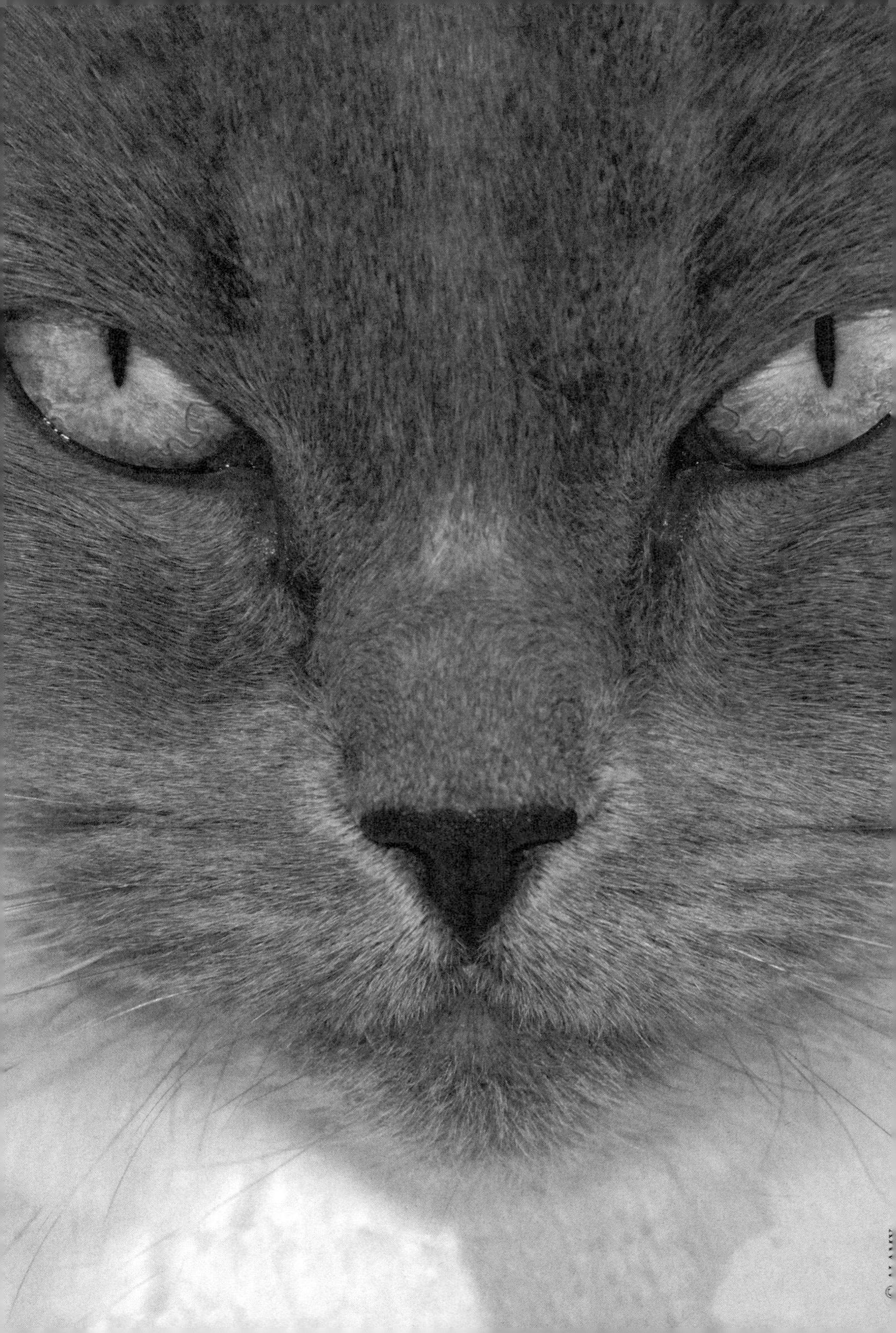

I am aware that according to present-day criteria, the story I am about to tell contains several shocking scenes which fall within the realms of sexual harassment and cruelty towards animals. A more lenient judge would at least mention inappropriate attitudes, male chauvinism, breach of trust and/or authority – all the terms one uses today for many good reasons and which I do not contest. However, this story is probably no more violent than it is erotic. Sorry. It appears to me to be sexual, but I'm not sure. In any case, it's true, down to the slightest detail, which is something after all.

It takes place in the mid-eighties, in a medium-sized city in the South of France. I had just begun my studies and I really liked my philosophy teacher, Mr Domino. Obviously, I've changed his name. Anyway, the poor man is dead now (I must point out straight away that I had nothing to do with it). 'Domino' isn't a bad choice for a pseudonym: it's close to his real one and has a ludic, philosophical side (the 'domino theory') to it. It also suggests, and I notice this as I'm writing, an idea of domination. But I regret that I'd surely disappoint the reader expecting bondage and sadomasochism. Mr Domino wasn't exactly the dominant male type.

So, Mr Domino had been through May '68. Which means a lot of things. For example, that he was both driven to despair and that he drank a lot. But he also threw cobblestones at policemen on the rue Gay-Lussac, and in spite of his receding hairline, pot belly and blotchy red face, we envied him his heroic period. It meant he had believed in a better world, in the possibility of dialogue between intellectuals and workers, in social justice, in organic goat's cheese, in world disarmament and in freedom of expression. And also in sexual freedom. I suppose.

Mr Domino, carried by the spirit of May '68, would sometimes give lessons in cafes, often treated his students as friends or even lovers, went about barefoot when it was hot enough, smoked in class and refused to give marks. I may as well say that today he'd be in prison. He was an excellent teacher. All I know about Rousseau, the Enlightenment, Hegel, Marx and also Lewis Carroll, I owe to him. Some of his sentences truly struck me, but he never played the guru. He was one of those people who listen to you as if you were saying something extraordinary, even at your most banal. He believed it didn't take much for a young human being, girl or boy, to choose to be free. But he was in despair. For a man like him, the eighties were hopelessly depressing. He had also fought in the Algerian War, before he threw cobblestones at policemen. Which is not an easy beginning for an existence.

Mr Domino supervised the *khôlles* from his own place. The *khôlles* is a French institution, an end-of-term oral exam. Although it is informal, it may determine whether or not you pass on to a higher level. It's stressful. Generally (no – not generally – always), you sit for it in a classroom, alone with the teacher. Today, I believe that such a tête-à-tête, even within the confines of a school building, would be perceived as extremely questionable. But Mr Domino preferred to give the *khôlles* from home, considering that since the student and teacher were obliged to sit through this stressful moment together, they may as well drink a beer and make themselves comfortable.

And so we made an appointment, which was simple enough, for noon one Saturday at his flat on rue Sainte-Blandine.

My morning had been complicated. I was used to smoking a substance which unfortunately was not freely sold, meaning I had to follow parallel economic routes to obtain a moderate quantity of it. That morning, since I didn't have the money necessary for the transaction, I had accepted the following arrangement: in exchange for the favour, I had committed myself to adopting a kitten. The friendly dealer's cat had indeed just given birth to seven kittens, and the good chap, panic-stricken, didn't know what to do with them.

And so there I was, a boarder who shared a room with two other girls, with a little cat that had just been weaned in my arms. Frankly, it was overpriced.

I don't know if the same applies in English, but *chat* and the feminine form *chatte* in French refer not only to the little domestic feline, but also to the female sex organs. Which explains why the audience laughs in Molière's famous play, *The School for Wives*, when the young and innocent Agnès announces to her father that 'the little cat is dead'.

In short. Walking to my *khôlle* exam, the little cat in my satchel, an idea had begun to form in my mind: make nice old Domino adopt the animal.

I rang the intercom downstairs. Domino invited me to come up. He lived on the fourth and final floor. I climbed the spiral staircase. I heard my name. I looked up. I saw a pink halo. Domino made a friendly gesture. He was leaning on the guardrail. He was completely naked.

From that point onwards my young brain had to deal with a combination of information which presented almost no common denominator. 1. I wanted my teacher to adopt my cat. 2. My teacher was completely naked. 3. I had to sit for an oral exam with him.

I was still only between the first and second floor. The cat was miaowing in my satchel. My teacher was leaning over. My brain was blocked. During the remaining two and a half flights of stairs, I recollected my thoughts and concentrated on the cat's adoption. My objective: behave as if everything were completely normal.

I held out my hand to the naked Domino. He shook it: Hello, how are you? His flat consisted of a large room furnished with a mattress, a rug and thousands of books piled up against the walls. We sat down on the rug. I freed the cat from my bag and explained my problem: I can't keep it. Would Mr Domino like to, let's say to start off with, take care of it? Uh, yes, answered Domino. I felt like I was taking advantage of the situation. But I was also terribly relieved.

The naked Domino, according to the ritual, held out the *khôlles* box to me: a mere cardboard box with subjects written on folded pieces of paper inside. I drew 'Rousseau and Freedom'.

I had twenty minutes to prepare my rundown. My teacher was sitting cross-legged in front of me and I was making an effort not to glance at his genitals. It was difficult. Rousseau and freedom. My retina was firmly imprinted with the pink, plump masses with whitish hairs that I had captured in my field of vision. Rousseau and freedom. The cat was miaowing. I asked if I could consult a book. I buried my nose in the sentences, pages and letters. After a long while my teacher offered me a coffee. The pink-and-white halo lifted itself up and walked towards the kitchen. Could you give the cat some milk? I asked. Uh, yes, answered Domino. Noise of an opening fridge. Gurgling of the coffee machine.

Outline in three parts. 1. Rousseau and the Natural Man. 2. The Conflict between Desire and the Law. 3. The Necessity of the Law.

'Are you ready?' Domino asked me. He used the familiar *tu* form, like he did with all his students. He sat back down in front of me. Coffee. I delivered my long-winded speech. Forty minutes – ten minutes per section, five minutes for the introduction, five minutes for the conclusion. It was long. 'All in all,' I said, 'there is no freedom without enlightened consent.' The cat miaowed. 'That's all very well,' said Domino. 'Very good. But what about the State?'

It was a bit of a blow for me. I had talked about the Law but not enough about the State. Even though Domino didn't give marks, this was going to be bad for my passing on to a higher level. '"When every man does as he pleases, he often does what displeases others, and this is not called a free state,"' quoted Domino, by heart and naked. I found the complete quote in *Letters Written from the Mountain*, and I read aloud: '"Freedom consists less in doing one's will than in not being submitted to the will of another; it consists also in not submitting someone else's will to one's own."' 'Oh yes,' commented a thoughtful Domino. I thereby reformulated my conclusion by expanding on the Revolution and French History, the country where freedom is fundamentally anti-libertarian. 'Very, very good,' sighed the naked Domino. 'Bravo.'

I stood up. Domino stood up. Things moved in the pink middle of his plump body. He opened his arms and stepped towards me, with U-shaped lips. He tried to place a funny kiss on my cheek. A cup of coffee was knocked over. 'Mr Domino,' I said without knowing what I was saying, 'I think you should really get dressed.' 'You do?' he hesitated, using the formal *vous* I had addressed him with. 'Yes,' I said. 'Very well,' he said. He rustled about in a corner, bent over between the piles of books. Two pink globes in the air, two short skinny legs. He found a pair of striped boxer shorts and put them on.

'Thank you for the cat, Mr Domino.' I shook his hand. He looked very melancholic. 'What cat?' he asked me. I pointed vaguely to the kitchen. I walked down the stairs. I didn't look back. In the spiral of the staircase I could perceive Domino, up above like a statue of pink salt, dressed in floppy underwear.

I spent the rest of the year avoiding Domino, and he trying to talk to me. Seen from the outside, or from the present day, we probably resembled a teacher and a student who were extremely embarrassed by a regrettable incident, the guilty teacher trying to excuse himself, the overwhelmed student fleeing the awful man. Whereas Mr Domino only wanted to give me back my lousy pussy, and I had no intention of taking it back. ■

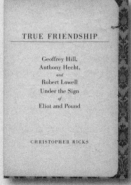

THE FIG TREE AND THE WASP

Brian Chikwava

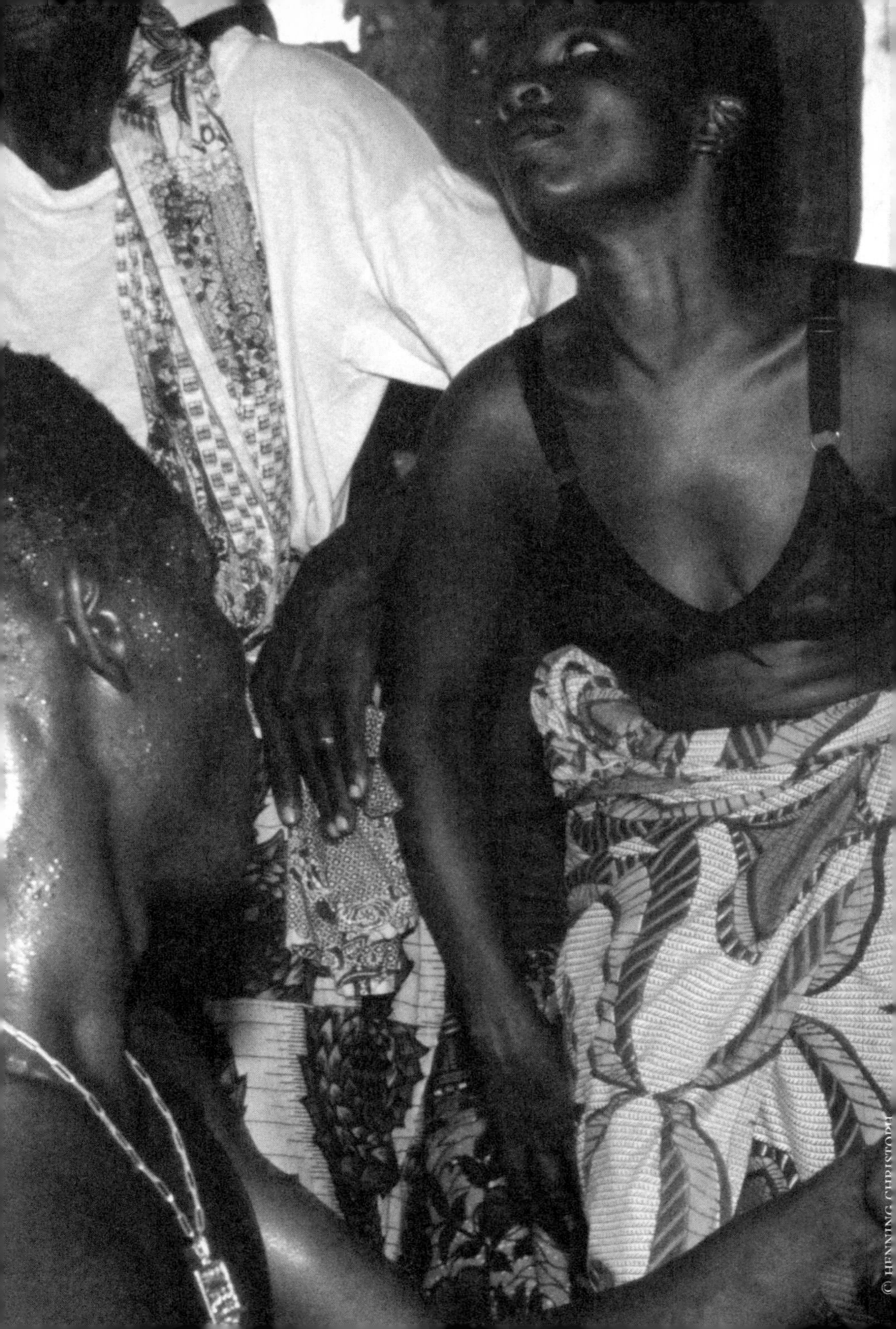

It was 1979 and I had just started primary school. That summer was the first time I witnessed what later became known as *iskokotsha*, a craze that would, in the euphoria of a newly independent Zimbabwe, trigger the focus of motion in popular dance to snake decisively, seductively, up the body, from the feet to the hips – a sex pantomime of outrageously suggestive moves that enthralled our young nation for the decade to come.

Being onomatopoeic, *iskokotsha* is derived partly from the beat of the snare-drum rim and the appropriate twirling of the body to that rhythm. The dance takes on a fuller character when understood by its other name, *kongonya*, which alludes to the carefree, if not contemptuously deliberate, rhythm in the gait of a large stubborn animal.

The day I first saw the dance was the day we had expected to end with the execution of my maternal grandfather.

Across the country and in my mother's home village of Monde, ten kilometres outside of Victoria Falls, the war was drawing to a conclusion and the principles and ideals of the guerrillas had become frazzled. Where they once asked villagers for food, they now made demands; where they had sought to operate by consent, they now issued ultimatums. On the military front, because the Rhodesian Army tortured and killed people for intelligence about them, the guerrillas' response came in the form of a blizzard of reprisals that were meant to keep communities silent. Soon entire villages were living in terror of both the army and the guerrillas. Their orders and demands were beyond questioning by then – at least that was how everyone understood it. Everyone except my grandfather.

He was only a week out of prison, having served ten years for collaborating with the guerrillas, and he must have been genuinely or wilfully unaware of the new order, or perhaps he was simply still possessed of an inmate's pointless recalcitrance. So when word was sent that it was the turn of the Mnkandla family and a few others to offer food towards the *pungwe* (the night-long rally that 'the boys' had called) and my grandfather sent back apologies that the family could not afford to give anything this time round, the stage was set for him to take the role of intransigent geriatric in the finest Nguni tradition.

The word that got back to the guerrillas was that there were some uncooperative families needing a 'gentle' reminder of how things were supposed to work. This was, after all, the Zimbabwe People's Revolutionary Army (ZIPRA) that was being slapped in the face.

A little less than an hour after my grandfather sent back the *mujibhas* (the young villagers who acted as scouts and messengers), half a dozen combatants accompanied by an equal number of *mujibhas* appeared on the brow of the hill that lay in front of the homestead. My uncle Elliot, also visiting with his wife at the time, got up to meet them amid a cacophony of dogs barking. On the veranda with us, my grandmother must have been regretting having let my grandfather have his way. A bit of beef or goat meat was not such a high price anyway, if the alternative was her husband's death.

By the time the half-dozen khaki-uniformed guerrillas got to the veranda, they were unequivocal in the pointing of their AK-47s. The old man was ordered to get up and head for the kraal, where they were going to make an example of him. He obliged and stood up, picking up his Tonga stool. He would not need it, he was told. But by now, having already switched to honest-to-goodness stubbornness, he refused to relinquish his seat. As he was led away, the grown-ups were probably already thinking of the aftermath, of picking up the pieces. My grandmother and mother had long ceased to respond to my little brothers' tugging and clinging to their frocks. Uncle Elliot, though probably feeling his bowels loosening, still had it in him to order the *mujibhas* away. They pretended to leave but scurried back to hide behind the log-wall granary, their faces occasionally poking out from behind a corner. They were ready to scamper across the hills to tell all that Munyatheli Mnkandla was finally finished.

After an endless hour during which everyone waited to hear the conclusive crack of an AK-47, we saw the guerrillas head back to the homestead. Their guns were slung across their backs, one of them was carrying my grandfather's stool while the other helped him totter along on his walking stick. This time they greeted my grandmother as sons of the house, offered their heartfelt apologies and handed back my grandfather's prison papers which they had requested half an hour earlier. In accordance with custom, the guerrillas introduced themselves, kinship was sought from both sides and it turned out that one of them shared the surname 'Maphosa' with my grandmother – she instantly became his aunt. Soon plans were afoot to relocate the *pungwe* to Mnkandla's home, but in the meantime the gramophone was taken out of the house and placed on the veranda.

Now, having loosened up, our new-found relations leapt into their dancing personas. On the turntable was a record which would lodge in my memory so that in the years to come, whenever I saw its zebra-emblazoned red label going round and round, I would be spun back to that afternoon. It was 'Jungle Jive', the township music hit number by Fast Fingers. Rifles slung across their backs and caps now tucked, half hanging out, into the rear pockets of their combat trousers, each of the guerrillas plunged into the music, quickly falling into rhythm with the constant knock of the snare drum and twirling the lower half of the body in the most suggestive and improper manner. At the front, what looked suspiciously like a small bag of onions jiggled through the khaki trousers, rocking the hips back, while at the rear a cap flapped, mischievously slapping the bum into the other court. The music, with its *kwela* pennywhistle origins, was not exactly the kind that went with *iskokotsha,* but its beat worked perfectly – or the combatants simply violated it into submission. And so in the dry, hot, motionless mid-afternoon air of Monde, 'Jungle Jive' was humped. Too embarrassed to watch this, my grandmother together with Uncle Elliot's wife, MaSibanda, and my mother cackled their way to the safety of the kitchen hut. Mnkandla, on his Tonga stool, watched his boys tilling the air as a grin verging on the undignified threatened to undo all his good work of the preceding hour.

The story has become tangled up with time, but family lore – variations of the story as told by Elliot – has it that the old man had played a high-stakes game that could easily have blown up in his face had his nerve failed. While being led to the tree that had been chosen as the site of his execution, his opening gambit had been to ask the guerrillas who their commander, or 'cwommander' as he pronounced it, was. He wanted to talk to their cwommander because now that they were executing him on the basis of malevolent hearsay, tomorrow the same hearsay would lead them unwittingly to execute their commander-in-chief, Joshua Nkomo, whom '… I left behind in jail paying a high price for you boys'.

Of course he had not been in the same jail as Nkomo, but that revelation and what must have been a perplexing absence of fear on the face of this pipe-sucking old fuck-up on his Tonga stool threw the would-be executioners off. The guerrillas lost their poise and said they had left their commander back where the *pungwe* was to be held. And so Mnkandla, a spirit medium and herbalist, reached for the initiative in the manner of a visiting grandfather plucking his expensive hat off the head of a badly brought up grandson who had snatched it off the old knee to start the game. Deploying the full oratory force of a venerable custodian of tradition, he put it to them that since their cwommander was on the other side of the village, he, Munyatheli Mnkandla, was by default presently their cwommander and was ordering them to leave a couple of their fellows guarding him, if need be, and to go and bring their cwommander here. Now! Soon, the law was laid down and an ethical order that had existed a decade earlier reimposed: freedom fighters operate in the area by consent, they do not make demands for food but accept whatever people can afford. And so followed the process of verifying who this peculiar old man was, culminating with the boys humping a *kwela* number in the screaming daylight.

Later that same year, soon after a ceasefire had been declared, we again visited my grandparents during the school holidays.

I had accompanied Cwommander Mnkandla and his smoking pipe on a walk around the village when we were called over by a group of guerrillas. Obviously still distrustful of the ceasefire, they were concealed behind thick foliage over which the canopy of a gnarly old fig tree hung still, swarmed by fig wasps and with the aroma of overripe figs tangible a good distance away. The guerrillas started off as expected: Is it OK on that side of the village? Who are those people who spent the night at the Moyo family homestead? As had now become customary, joviality followed: Come on, spare us some of that tobacco of yours, old man. My grandfather could command from the guerrillas a degree of the deference reserved for elders but not enough to stop them getting distracted by the occasional maiden strolling serenely down the path with a bucket of water or firewood on her head, pretending to have seen nothing because to see something then had come to mean being a potential witness, a burden that still held the whiff of death. On the part of the guerrillas, probably sex-starved and certainly driven by procreative urges after years of living amid death, the temptation to wolf-whistle was apparent but resisted – carelessness could see comrades perish.

And so followed a spell in which my grandfather had to fend off questions about talismans for luring girls. He protested, saying what they were looking for was something that only Malawians and other exotic peoples knew how to do. As pointed as their bayonets, the carnal desires of these young men, who out of necessity had spent years living beyond the reach of their traditional social norms, would shape those of the nation.

We departed with a handful of figs which, on our way back home, my grandfather eagerly introduced me to. Two decades later, I would come to know about the uniqueness of the fig tree. Over millennia, the fig tree has developed a co-evolutional relationship with the fig wasp: the wasp cross-pollinates the plant and can only perpetuate itself through the plant's fruit. The female wasp lays its eggs inside a fig, the eggs hatch and the larvae develop into adults. The females, who are winged, do not possess the big jaws required to gnaw their way out of the fruit, while the males, who possess tearaway jaws, are wingless. At this point a dubious compromise is struck: each male tunnels his way to the skin of the fruit and then crawls back to lead the female up the new tunnel, but before she can escape completely, he grabs her in a final desperate act of coitus, deposits his seed and then, exhausted, allows her to fly away. With all the females having escaped to lay their eggs elsewhere and propagate the species, the fig fruit rots and, at the whisper of a breeze, obligingly breaks loose and plunges down to earth, taking the male wasps with it.

In 1980, when Rhodesia became Zimbabwe, the country woke to the full impact of the cultural tremors that had flattened much of sub-Saharan Africa: the boys and girls from the *bhundu* (the bush), as the guerrillas were called, brought *iskokotsha* from their training grounds in Zambia, Tanzania and Mozambique. A new way of being had arrived. They emerged from the *bhundu* hot-stepping to the Zambian copper-belt sounds of Dr N. P. Kazembe & his Super Mazembe, Tanzania's Orchestra Super Mazembe and others – all of them mutations of Cuban rumba-inspired sounds from the Congos.

These ex-combatants revelled in being strangers among their own people: on the street, at the beer garden or in the shebeen. Here they were, with a glint of danger, revolution and a new exoticism from north of the Zambezi. The way they moved on the dance floor made people sit up – they had to decipher this language, to learn new ways. You are one thing today and then, in this new tomorrow, as old notions of the self fall away like masks of mud-cake and turn to dust, you are something else, someone else. At least that seemed to be the case. *Iskokotsha* arrived and people found, to their amazement, that they too could do it; it seemed inconceivable that beyond pantomime, words would be necessary. With *iskokotsha*, faces would light up with recognition, yet no one could actually name what it was that they recognized. Then again maybe, with hindsight, people left unmentioned what they recognized here because, as the girls walking past us and the guerrillas by that fig tree had made clear:

whatever had the shadow of death behind it, we pretended not to see. We could not be witnesses. We had, in Zimbabwe, found a way of acting out our sexual urges but not a way of talking about the more difficult questions around sex, my mother would say a few years later. By then the dance had taken on a life of its own and was now a far cry from its freedom-fighter origins.

In early 1982, my father had just been promoted to officer-in-charge and transferred to head a police station in the small town of West Nicholson. The family had to uproot and follow him. The country was caught in an exhilarating maelstrom of change and myth-making: Zimbabwe had been delivered, the nation was free. Salisbury had become Harare, Essexvale became Esigodini, Victoria Falls briefly became Mosi-oa-Tunya before reverting back to Victoria Falls, and each guerrilla made a personal decision whether or not to shed his or her *nom de guerre*. My family, not to be left out, soon had an American pit bull named Marx. That was when, for the first time, the blur of hip motion that was *iskokotsha* came into our house, brought by our new housemaid, Silingiwe, much to the consternation of my mother who made it clear she did not want to see 'that kind of thing' in the house.

It is probably accurate to say that it was in 1982 that I became aware of the potential of *iskokotsha* as shorthand for social survival. Silingiwe was capable of displaying near Victorian propriety one minute and being impossibly exhibitionist the next. She would be the most proper maid in front of important guests, but as she got to know the family better there would be those times when in the kitchen, with my mother out of sight, she would show my brothers and me, in exaggeratedly slow motion, the techniques behind *iskokotsha*: legs astride and back arched in a posture that short-circuited my adolescent brain and rendered me mute. Her hips would turn into a riveting kinetic spectacle as the snappy sounds of a Four Brothers' tune urged her into taking the horse-riding position on an imaginary pleasure chair, surrendering in absolute abandonment to that primitive delight that reaches its pinnacle in the spellbinding stretch of music where the essential elements in both song and dancer are revealed: the song is pared down to the staccato rhythm of the snare drum and a hypnotic snaking guitar line, while the dancer, no longer of this world, pulsates to a most naked instinct. In this way, she would later find street cred in the eyes of my mother and her friends.

Surrounded by ranches and gold mines, West Nicholson was a small town organized around the canning and mining industries – canned beef, Fray Bentos, Oxo and gold were what it produced and freighted to the rest of the country. Culturally it punched way above its weight, attracting virtually every significant band or musician in the country. It was here, in the beer gardens, shebeens and community halls, where the legend of a young man popularly known as 'Screw Vet' was whispered. This was someone to whom even Silingiwe sat up and paid attention when he took to the dance floor.

Screw Vet was in his early twenties. He was one of the groundsmen at West Nicholson Primary School (where my brothers and I were enrolled) and blessed with an athletic body sculptured by manual labour. Had he had enough in his wardrobe to choose from, he would have been a dandy. As it was, most of the time he was seen in his gumboots, a white vest tucked into his flannel trousers which in turn were unfailingly tucked into his boots. This was his trademark outfit throughout the year. He took great care with his trousers – they were always immaculately ironed, with a crease on each leg sharp enough to sever in two any fly that made the mistake of landing on them.

People were mildly amused and took him for an eccentric and semi-literate young manual labourer. But all of this is not why Screw Vet made an indelible mark on my memory. Obsessive about his looks, affected and semi-literate as he was, when it came to what mattered – *iskokotsha* – Screw Vet was peerless.

The beer gardens and shebeens were the domain of many Screw Vets and Silingiwes, the young men and women who worked as housemaids, gardeners and cooks or at the factory, who lived for their end-of-month pay packages and the chance to unburden themselves at the local joint or shebeen. At the beer hall, the patrons drank traditional beer while the jukebox delivered the tunes. Down the road, the shebeen queen spun sounds off her gramophone and served bottled beer – either way, the gyrating patrons were only a solicitous wiggle of the hips from getting their claws on the object of their desires while those with less coordinated bodies suffered a social death. And in that way the new pop slogan, *yekel' omunye wena uzamdabulela!* – 'let go of the other or you'll ruin his/her clothes!' – was heard on the radio and, later, 'Wapenga Nayo Bonus', the Four Brothers' hit that encapsulated the monetary and moral extravagance that went with pay days. It was here, in these places of excess, when nature turned and its curse fell like a scythe on these young lives, that the fate of a fig wasp would seem an infinitely better alternative. For in the fig-wasp world, when all the girls have flown away to lay their eggs elsewhere and propagate the species, the fig fruit only goes down with the boys. In the world of men, when the rot set into the compounds and townships, it spared neither sex. Big jawed or winged, they all came down in the silent darkness of their fruit.

Because *iskokotsha* took hold in the rural population long before it found a following in the urban areas, it was often portrayed as a particularly bawdy rural aberration. Dance was supposed to be charming. But more often people were torn between surrendering to the possibilities of self-discovery that the new dance held or dismissing it as the preserve of people with no self-control. At least that seemed to be the case with my mother and the new friends she was making in West Nicholson, especially when Silingiwe took to showing off her talents in front of them. A line had to be drawn somewhere.

Usually my mother would invite her friends to our house and they would spend the afternoon in the gazebo, drinking tea and making womanly talk. It was probably the eagerness to see these new friendships blossom that made her plant a wireless radio on the table. This is how Silingiwe ended up there among these women. She would take a shawl, roll it up and tie it around her waist – accentuating the gyrations of her hips. When it got to the part of the song where she had to go down on a beat, she would trigger shrieks of disgusted delight among the women. The spectacle of Silingiwe seemingly grinding her crotch onto an imaginary figure famously had MaNcube, the only smoker among the women, lighting the wrong end of her cigarette. Fracture their ribs with laughter as they may have done, what each of them recognized in the dance was never something to be put into words.

With time, my mother, a nurse, became concerned for Silingiwe's health – the picture coming out of the hospital wards was bleak: these were stories of once robust neighbours now reduced to skeletal shadows of themselves. The deep-lying natural rhythms of existence – of people begetting children by whom they would be buried at the end of their lives – were fractured. This illness took no account of that tradition. Now, even the rising and setting of the sun seemed uncertain as parents grew accustomed to burying their children.

And since the general attitude was to avoid HIV tests – the rationale being that a bad result could deprive you of your happy-go-lucky spirit – this was only the tip of the iceberg, epidemiologists warned. The fashionable euphemisms that now crowded the condolence columns of newspapers were of state functionaries or prominent businesspeople dying of 'a long illness', 'pneumonia', 'meningitis' and 'tuberculosis'. The preceding years had allowed a new freedom – if you caught an STD, you got treated at the hospital and came back to play. The popular refrain among the young women then was '… I don't suck a lollipop that's still inside a wrapper', meaning that a condom was simply a non-starter. This had also been one of Silingiwe's favourite battle cries as she threw herself at some tune during the day, when my parents were at work. But when it came to talking about the new disease which, unlike gonorrhoea or syphilis, could not be treated, my mother complained that Silingiwe simply clammed up. It was then that my mother said we had in Zimbabwe found a way of acting out our sexual fantasies but not a way of talking about sexual health. I guess if my mother had had her way, public health policy in the 1980s would have revolved around talking, talking and more talking until people were at ease talking about sex. But instead of conversation, the devastation of those unprecedented deaths coming so soon after our liberation seemed to have us all in the grip of a national seizure. Our old selves, cast off, had turned to dust and no longer afforded us refuge. Any chance of survival rested on learning new ways and training our tongues to articulate what had, by consensus, until now, remained taboo.

The leisure centre in West Nicholson was a large estate comprising the community hall, the beer hall, the outdoor cinema and the sports field. This was where the rituals of the new nation were enacted: official holidays marking, in turn, Independence Day, Heroes Day, Africa Day, Workers Day. My father was normally the point man for the government officials who came to address the crowd on these occasions. And of course we, my mother and the rest of us, were expected to attend.

The ceremonies started mid-morning with a grand speech, usually followed by a police and army display. Sometimes the air force would fly by in Alouette helicopters and thrill the crowds with re-enacted battle manoeuvres. Then there would be free food and beer for everyone and a football match followed by a band concert in the community hall. Here, the celebrated Screw Vet would reveal the full orbital range of his magic: gumboots, white vest and trousers with their famous fly-wasting blades. He would walk across the dance floor and the entire hall would erupt.

These were days when waiting for a concert to start was like waiting for the rains – the concert time on the poster only served as an indicator but when the band would actually appear onstage was anyone's guess. Meanwhile, someone would be spinning records through the PA system, and because people were quite intoxicated by then, these warm-up exercises easily degenerated into full-scale contests with people challenging each other on the dance floor.

We had heard that he could dance, but to me and my family Screw Vet was just the slightly odd groundsman at my school who, due to concerns about snakes, occasionally came to drive us away from the mulberry orchard. But here in the community hall, as we waited for the band, Screw Vet, in that disinterested and enigmatic manner of immense talents, waved the crowd away and prowled towards the exit, not to be seen again until the concert was in full swing. When he reappeared the hall swelled with anticipation, clearing the way for him. Screw Vet was transformed from dandy wheelbarrow pusher to eminent star. This time he would do his thing to a cover of 'Shauri Yako', Orchestra Super Mazembe's sprawling hit number that offered ample scope for anyone to transport themselves beyond the horizons that hemmed in everyday life. When he stamped his authority on his territory, it was with awe-inspiring grace and style that his hips swirled, syncopated by singularly coarse and wilful stabs. Perhaps only on his waist lay the possibility of a hulahoop being held in a blur of infinite motion. The techniques that we had known from Silingiwe took on another character and even she would sit still and watch because with Screw Vet it suddenly dawned on you that it is not the size of the swing that you put into the hips that mattered but the hip that you put into the swing, the cool that was inscribed in its many variations into the dance – the impatient lover's backward throw of the head, the oversexed brute rocking around with an imaginary female impaled on his phallus, the considerate lover grinding down his hips with staggering care.

At the end of the song Screw Vet would get his white hanky out of his pocket, wipe his forehead with a flourish and vanish, leaving the men and older women shaking their heads, the nubile chasing after him, and the band picking up the pieces of their concert. Screw Vet demonstrated the power of *iskokotsha* to deliver women at his feet and the cynics whispered from the margins: Yah! All those women. How long before we hear that this boy excavated his grave with his penis?

In 1989 Cwommander Mnkandla died. This was also the year my family left West Nicholson for Esigodini where we would live briefly before finally moving back to Bulawayo. Silingiwe stayed behind in West Nicholson and we all missed her, speculating about what she could be possibly be doing with her life, whether she was well. Of course this kind of speculation invariably extended to Screw Vet in some shape or form, never mind that we did not know him personally. And some of those concerns about Silingiwe and Screw Vet were ones that we dared not dwell on for too long lest we jinxed them. They were creatures of that era and perhaps instead of impotent concern for their future, one way to honour their memory and let go would have been to turn to Richard Francis Burton: 'We dance along Death's icy brink, / but is the dance less full of fun?'

By that year, every town in the country had its urban legends of shebeen girls who went about helping themselves to other women's husbands; tired tales of promiscuous men who contracted the incurable disease elsewhere and brought the illness home to their spouses. It looked as if that era was on its way out. But there were, presumably, shenanigans going on at Esigodini Police Station and for some reason my father's secretary decided to do my mother a favour, calling her to say that one of the other secretaries in the office had her eye on my father. She was young, my father's secretary, just the other side of twenty-five. What she had not counted on was that my mother did not believe that people would do her favours for no apparent reason. Profanities that I never thought my mother capable of uttering issued from my parents' bedroom that evening, but the roof of the house held down. My mother prevailed. In the morning she asked my father to bring his secretary home with him after work. Once the poor girl had been delivered, my mother took her to the master bedroom. My father's brother was visiting then and I was with him when my father, visibly shaken, came to join us in the lounge.

After about half an hour my mother emerged from the bedroom, went out to the garden and came back not with a stick, but what looked like an entire tree. My father and his brother knew better than to try to stop her. And so she set about working on the unfortunate girl. My father's secretary was obviously the sort who internalized things, expressing neither pain nor pleasure. Still, sporadic moans and yelps could be heard. It was supposed to be some variation of tough love, at least those were the cultural pretensions, but you knew that victim and torturer had swapped roles and that thankfully there were no electrodes or such instruments lying about in the house.

My father became increasingly jittery. He begged his brother to go and intervene; being a guest he stood a chance of being respected, but even he was not quite sure how to handle my mother and turned to me instead: 'B., can't you go and stop your mother? She'll hurt her.' This would have been funny if not for the fact that someone was having it bad in there. Me trying to stop my mother was a laughable proposal – she would dismiss me with a single contemptuous glare. Eventually my father gathered the courage to rescue the young lady and she was in a state when she emerged. At least my mother had restricted herself to the girl's legs, and so her stockings looked almost magnificent, in that other way.

In the lounge, this being no time to open a cold bottle of beer, my father, tireless music collector that he was, went down to sit on the floor by the hi-fi – the spot on which he had spent many evenings lying with his headphones on while his supper went cold, much to the irritation of my mother. As he and his brother fumbled about for conversation, he flipped through his collection, putting aside his old favourites: Victoria Jazz Band, Wendo Kolosoy, Grand Kallé, Docteur Nico and Tabu Ley. Then he started playing them one after another until he tired, sat on the sofa and left Victoria Jazz Band to play on again and again: one of those numbers that, like the Zambezi, starts off shallow, turns and meanders at length while the snare drum obligingly counts each yard, goes through rapids, down the falls, acquires ferocious energy, twirls and narrows as it eats its way through rock, assumes still and trembling depths, and finally, its murderous urge ebbing away, widens up and flows gently into a larger body of water. At least such was the sense of calm when a few hours later my mother and father, emotionally exhausted, lay on opposite sofas fast asleep while my uncle smoked a cigarette and I played with my brothers in the garden. Maybe for my family it was then that the curtain came down on the preceding decade, with my parents at ease with each other and the memories of Cwommander Mnkandla, Silingiwe, Screw Vet and the legacy of *iskokotsha* gently floating away into the larger pool of human experience. ■

POEM | ANNE CARSON

Hang It Up

hang up your blood cell phone mr white slaver
hang it up, we're all here
the police is here
the former government is here
the new revolutionary government is here
science is here
poetry is here
the dictionary is here
jazz and its history are here
charity is here
the major food groups are here
the major museums are here
the urchins are here
all arguments for the existence of god are here
trance is here
negritude is here
the surrealists are here
the ice cream is here
a clash of ethnographies is here
sad choirs are here
dust is here
the changing names of the oceans are here
summer is here with its accelerations inside a big slowness
the siege, the sack and the ransack are here
the swirling behind the lip

is here, the back biscuits
the tent of sleep
the plan to hurt it all
the plan to hurt hawks
the wild hawk caress
the dizzy sky and on
the foam on the neck and on
the eating
the raping
the dandelions
the churning hip, her corrupt hip
her butter gears
the awful rocking
the work shed
the shed smell
the clear rib, clear all, clear sweethearts
the animal char *stalag*
the snow after, the snow in the weeds
the *Come shadow come* the Take this shadow up
we have enough girls
we have enough pills
we know who is 'it'
they have their little shovels
there is no one to call
hang up your blood cell phone mr white slaver
hang it up

THE SPA

Tom McCarthy

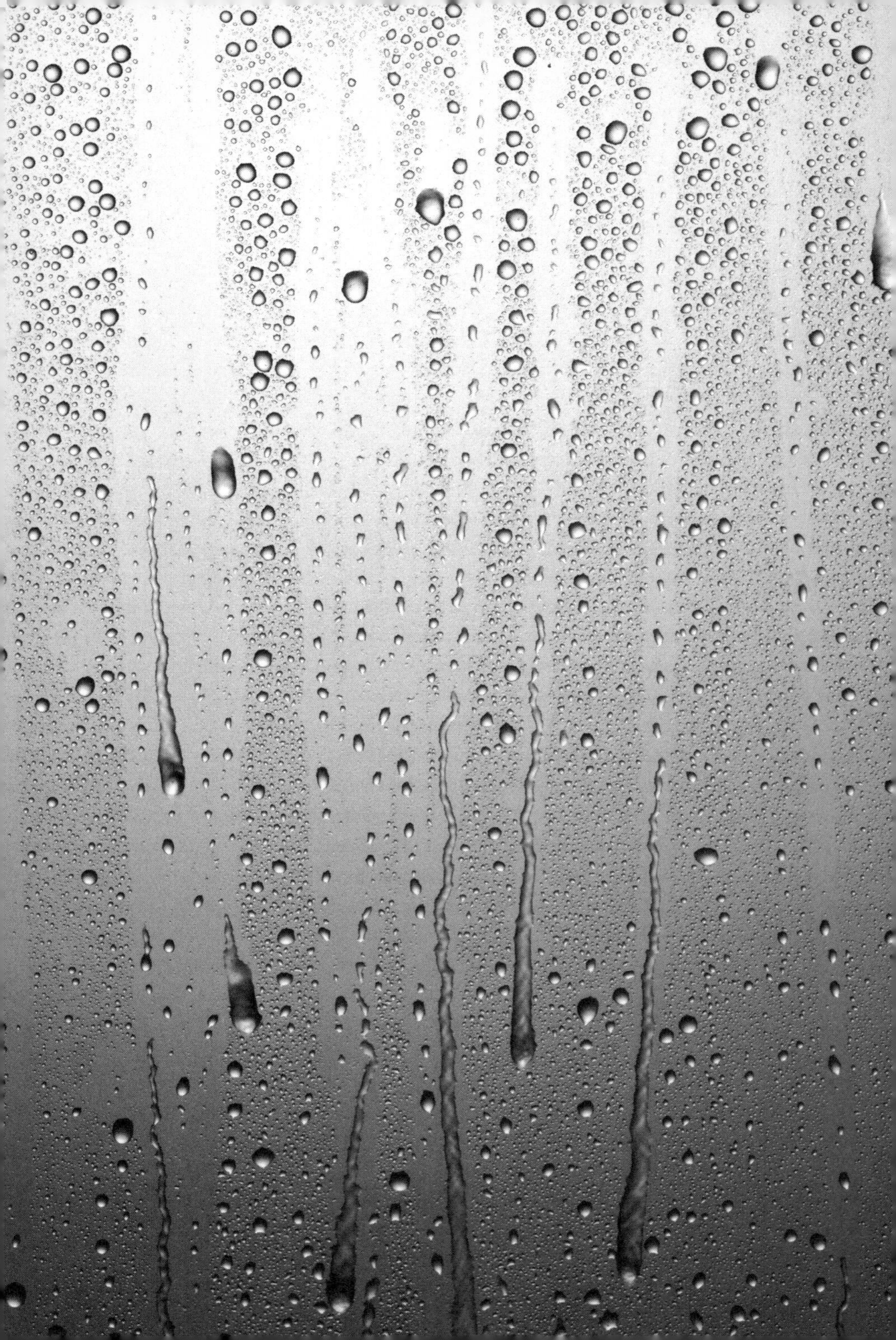

I

Klodĕbrady is a twenty-three-hour journey from Portsmouth; from Versoie, twenty-eight. Serge and Clair board first a train, then a boat, then another grand train laid on by the International Sleeping Car Company and, finally, when this pulls up somewhere near Dresden, a series of smaller trains that carry them across borders of countries, time zones, principalities and semi-autonomous regions Serge has never even heard of. If the names sliding across the compartment's window beside telegraph poles, red-roofed farmhouses and haystacks that seem to float ten feet above the ground seem vaguely familiar to him, this probably owes more to the fairy tales Maureen would tell him as a child than to anything he's learned from Clair of geography or history. He's passed through zones of boredom and exhaustion too, emerged from them and started waking up now for the journey's last leg. His senses, though out of kilter, are alert; the lethargy that's hung above him like a pall for months seems to have lifted – not completely, but a little: lifted and lightened.

The train's come to a stop. It's not a station: they're just waiting for a signal to change, or a point to switch, or an instruction to be shouted from the trackside in a foreign language. Serge stands up, pulls the top half of the window down, leans out and looks around. It's the end of summer: bushes and trees beside the lines are overgrown and faded; dandelions and weeds stand a foot tall between the sleepers. The countryside is flat. A mile or two away, a smokestack seems to rise straight from it. Nearer by, an earthworks plant groans as its stilted runways convey ballast before dropping it on to a growing mound. Other, fully grown mounds of the stuff stretch for hundreds of yards beside the railway line, strangely black against the blue sky and golden foliage.

'It's the cysteine,' Clair says, noticing Serge looking at the mounds.

'Sistine? Like the chapel?'

'No, what makes it black: the chemical. Cysteine and sulphur, chloride, sodium, what have you. That's what's going to cure you.'

He tosses Serge a brochure from among the papers lying beside him on the bench seat. The train's almost empty; with the compartment to themselves, they've spread out. Serge lets the brochure land on his own bench seat, then sits down again and picks it up. The front cover bears a drawing of an elegant lady strolling with a parasol along a boulevard lined with Graeco-Roman buildings, a glass in her hand. Beneath this image's border and slightly in front of it due to the perspective adopted by the brochure's illustrator, a large red heart is held aloft by a jet of water while a cherub, balancing above the heart on one foot, breaks across the border into the main picture to strew roses across the lady's path. Above the lady's parasol, shot through with black sunrays, are the words 'Kloděbrady Baths'.

The accompanying text gives the town's history, which seems to consist of a series of invasions, wars and squabbles over succession. One such squabble, dwelt on at some length by the brochure's author, sees the heirs of a King Mstislav accusing the pretender to his throne, one Vladimir, of poisoning their father, only for it to turn out that he'd died of 'corruption of the blood due to bad humour' – a cue for Vladimir, cleared of foul play, to decapitate his libellers. This Mstislav, or perhaps another, is mentioned a few paragraphs later, only now the humour has become a *tumour*: he (or his namesake) it was, the brochure says, who, 'seeking for his way in the labyrinth of events and social problems' prior to his blood's corruption, established Kloděbrady as a centre for 'radical social oppinions' – laying the ground for the progressive reign of the man who, emerging eighty or so years later, would eventually become the town's saint, Prince Jiři.

'This is interesting,' Serge says. 'This engineer, Maxbrenner, had to lay pipes beneath the whole town, leading out from under the castle, in order to create the spa. He plumbed in pumps, and heaters, and all sorts of things. So now, it says here, "all visitors may divertize themselves imbibing of the restorative balm." Oh, look: here's a list of what it's got in it.'

His eye runs down a table in which cysteine breaks down into sulphur, which in turn subdivides into various chlorides, carbonates and sulphates: chloride of sodium, chloride of lithium, of potassium; chloride, sulphate and carbonate of magnesium; carbonate of lime; then, intriguingly, 'free and easily liberated' types of carbonic acid. The heaviness inside Serge's stomach that's a constant presence for him these days makes itself felt as he reads the table. He flips the page and finds a photograph of Kloděbrady's Grand Hotel, its terraces alive with water-swilling people, flags of all the states of Europe fluttering above them and, above these, the heart-and-cherub logo once again.

The logo's waiting for them at the station, painted on the wood beside the town's name, its heart blackened by grime. Porters load their bags on to a trolley and push this, rattling, up the main drag. There are nurses, chattering in groups of three or pushing wheel-chaired cripples past kiosks selling trinkets and chemists' shops above whose doors hang model scales with snakes coiled around them.

The Grand Hotel's terraces are half empty. Chairs are leaned up against tables. The porters hand Serge and Clair over to their counterparts in the hotel, who take them to their rooms. In his, Serge finds, beside the bed, a season ticket to the baths and two bottles of sparkling but slightly murky-looking water. There's also a menu of the therapies on offer, with a list of prices: inhalation, twenty-nine crowns; gas injection, twenty crowns fifty; underwater massage, twenty-two; and so on.

Dinner is at seven. The long dining room has a bar at one end, behind which a white-coated waiter stands, hands on the counter, bottles rising up from staggered shelves like organ pipes behind him. The room's just under half full. Serge and Clair are seated by another waiter at a small round table and served quail and boiled potatoes with a bottle of red wine.

'Drink it slowly,' Clair says. 'It's supposed to be good for digestion.'

Serge shrugs. The other diners glance their way occasionally while speaking a mishmash of languages. Serge can pick out French, German and Spanish; Clair identifies Hungarian, Serbian and Russian on top of these. English is spoken as well, but, exchanged as a currency of convenience between people to whom it's not native, sounds foreign too. After dinner, while they're taking coffee in a lounge whose walls are lined with local wildlife specimens – otters, eels, pikes, water rats and toads – stuffed behind slightly darkened glass, a German man comes up and, introducing himself to them as Herr Landmesser, asks them what they're 'in for'.

'It's the boy,' says Clair. '*Das Kind.* Stomach complaints. Me, I'm as right as rain.'

'If you can say that, you are a lucky man,' Herr Landmesser answers with a deep, sardonic laugh. 'Or happily ignorant. Which doctor will you see?'

'Dr Filip,' answers Serge. 'My first appointment is tomorrow morning.'

'My doctor also, Filip. Gout, for me.' Herr Landmesser points down at his foot. 'For Filip, it is all the same: all moral.'

Serge begins to ask him what he means but is cut off by the arrival in their group of a tallish, middle-aged lady.

'So young!' she says in a grainy voice as she looks at Serge. 'I have a niece so young as you. You should meet her, when you would be in Rotterdam one day. Me, I have heart problems. How long will you stay here?'

'Three weeks, I think.' Serge looks at Clair to confirm this, but Clair seems too offended, or worried, by Herr Landmesser's jibe to take part in the conversation.

'*Pani!*' the tallish, middle-aged lady calls out to a waiter who's just passed by with a coffee pot. He doesn't hear her, so she sets out after him. Herr Landmesser, too, moves away from them towards some bookshelves. Clair and Serge sit for a little longer in depleted silence, then retire upstairs. Serge drifts off to the sound of running water not far from the hotel, a stream his mind makes flow again internally, recasting it as dark, with creatures moving slowly through it.

II

He wakes up early, some time before Clair, takes a light breakfast, then wanders along the paths that join the small domed mausoleums to each other in the park. An orchestra is playing beside one, in a bandstand. As he approaches it he realizes that the seated musicians are arranged in a heart shape; also that the mausoleums are in fact not mausoleums: they're pavilions housing fountains. People stroll from one to the next, holding their glasses out beneath the jets until they're full, then slowly sipping as they move on. A group of kaftaned Jews with beards and side curls chat in Polish and Yiddish as they drink; two Russians talk to one another loudly, gargling and spitting between sentences.

Serge doesn't have a glass. He cups his hands and holds them out into the fountain. The water's not particularly cold and, bizarrely, doesn't feel particularly *wet* either. It's got a kind of sooty feel to it. He draws his hands up to his face and looks at it: it's cloudy, slightly dark, with bubbles in it. He takes a sip: it's cloudy-tasting too, and a little bitter. A nurse wanders up and says something he doesn't understand. He raises his shoulders and looks blankly back at her; she makes a drinking-from-glass gesture with her hand, and points towards a kiosk selling glasses of the same slightly opaque quality as the wildlife cases in the hotel's lounge. Beside it, a signpost's arrows bear four names, each painted in large capitals: MIR, MAXBRENNER, ZAMACEK, LETNA. None of them say GRAND HOTEL, but Serge manages to find his way back there by following the same drag he walked up with the porters yesterday, past the trinket-selling kiosks and the chemists with their scales and snakes.

He finds Clair waiting agitated for him on the terrace.

'Your appointment's in five minutes. Hurry up!'

'I'm ready,' Serge shrugs back.

They head in the opposite direction from the fountains, past a statue of a crowned horseman and a large building up and down whose steps columns of nurses move, until they arrive at a smaller building.

Here, beside the front door, is a plaque with the name FILIP and a string of letters on it. Inside, a receptionist directs them to a waiting room. Several other patients are sitting in this, most of them holding jars half full of some sort of dark, silky material: they're the same size as the ones Bodner stores the honey in at Versoie, with the same bronze screw-on lids. After a few minutes Serge's name is called.

'Do you want me to come in with you?' Clair asks.

'No,' answers Serge.

Dr Filip is a small man with unkempt white hair and a stringy beard and whiskers. From behind thin, steel-rimmed spectacles, his eyes fix Serge with a disapproving look. Around him, tables, trays and treadmills are arrayed like the musical instruments of some outlandish orchestra. Strangest of all is a large machine that takes up a whole bench. Its cogs and filaments conjoin parts that look like they belong to printing presses, breweries or miniature railways. In its central segment, a dome the same shape as the fountain pavilions rises up, a spiral staircase carrying a copper cable from its apex down its side and on towards a fuse to which it's soldered.

'Carrefax, with *C*, not *K*,' says Dr Filip. 'Sit down.'

Instinctively, Serge looks around the room for his father before realizing that 'Carrefax' means him and complying with Dr Filip's order.

'Notes from English doctor indicate chronic intestinal problems,' Dr Filip continues. His voice is sharp, and seems to issue from the tiniest of apertures nestled among the whiskers. 'Please to describe them.'

Serge sticks his hands beneath his thighs and shuffles in his chair. 'It's like a big ball in my stomach,' he says. 'A big ball of dirt.'

'Why you say "dirt"?' asks Dr Filip.

'Well, because it's dark. It seems that way.'

'You having constipation?'

Serge nods, reddening.

'And lethargy?'

'Yes,' Serge says. 'Very much.'

'Headache?'

'Also.'

'Please to lie on table. But first remove shoes and shirt.'

Serge slides his shirt and shoes off and climbs up on to the table. Dr Filip pushes Serge's shoulders down into its flannel-covered surface with cold hands which then move to Serge's stomach, tapping as though sounding a box or wall. Serge begins to speak but Dr Filip cuts him off.

'Shh …'

He holds his hand over Serge's midriff and, tapping it a few more times – gently, as though nudging a dial – lowers his head and listens.

'Not good,' he says after a while. 'A blockage. Stagnant. You are having autointoxication. Skin is dark, eyes too. You seeing well, or not?'

'Not,' Serge says. 'I mean no. It's kind of …'

'How is?' Dr Filip asks, impatient.

'Furry.'

'What is meant?'

'Furry, like fur. The hair of animals. Small hairs. It's like …'

His voice trails off.

Dr Filip says: 'Please to provide a sample.'

'Sample of what?' Serge asks.

'Stool,' Dr Filip answers. His cold hands pull Serge's shoulders upright and turn them towards a low chair with a hole in its seat and a kidney-shaped tray beneath it.

'I can't,' Serge says.

'Not to be embarrassed,' Dr Filip sneers disdainfully.

'It's not that,' Serge explains, reddening again. 'I mean I can't. It doesn't want to …'

'You speak of what "it" wants?' Dr Filip's stringy eyebrows climb up towards his hairline, and his glasses ride up with them. 'So: I am arranging enema for you this afternoon. Also,' he continues, turning to his desk and picking up a pen, 'I am giving you diet from which not to digress. Lactose: soured milk and cereal. And fruit. No meat. You give this to hotel kitchen; they will administer.' He hands Serge two cards. 'And you will follow hydrotherapy course. Here is schedule.' He slides from a drawer a sheet of paper and, reaching behind him, pulls from a shelf a honey jar, then passes both these to Serge. 'Please to go now.

Return tomorrow afternoon at four. Also drink constantly the water.'

Serge walks back to the hotel holding the jar, wondering what he's meant to do with it. He tries to hand it in with his menu card, but the maître d' returns it to him, instructing him to take it to his next appointment, which turns out to be in the building that he saw the nurses entering and leaving. The nurse Serge sees, in a room sharp from disinfectant, makes him lower his trousers and pants and bend across another segmented table whose lower end is ramped down to the ground; then she inserts a rubber tube in him and turns a tap on. The warmish water enters and then leaves him, carrying no more than a small fragment of whatever's in him out with it.

'You have bottle?' she asks.

'Bottle?' Serge says. 'No. Should I?'

'Doctor has give you one, I think …'

The honey jar. 'I didn't realize that was meant for …'

'I use another,' she says. 'Show me card.'

He shows it to her. She copies his name and number on to a small piece of paper and hands the card back to him.

A sharpness that the enema has somehow lent his vision stays with him for a while: the air around the park as he walks back through it seems brighter, clearer and less flecked. The feeling lasts for an hour or so; then the world veils back up. As he heads to his bedroom after a dinner of soured milk and what looks like horse food, he passes the stuffed otters, eels and pikes, and realizes that he should have compared his vision, when describing it to Dr Filip, to the glass of their cases: it has the same clouded quality, the same fine-filamented graininess as everything he sees.

The hydrotherapy begins the next morning. After a fruit-and-yogurt breakfast and a wander round the Mir fountain with a glass purchased from the kiosk by the signpost, he visits the complex in which hydrotherapy is offered. It's the Maxbrenner building, built, like the Letna one in which he got his enema yesterday, around the spring whose name it bears. Serge presents his card at the front desk, and is ushered on towards the building's innards. A musty smell fills its corridors; the air itself is moist and sulphurous. Opening the door of the room he's been directed to, he's attacked by vapour which invades his nostrils and half scalds his lips. Inside, against a wall, are rows of cabinets, large escritoires with hinged covers. Some of these are open; others, closed, contain men, locked inside them with only their heads protruding from the top like unsprung jack-in-the-boxes. Other men's heads jut out horizontally from blankets wrapped tightly round their bodies as they lie on benches, steaming. They look like insects, like pupating larvae lifted from boiling water.

A nurse takes Serge's card and leads him first to a changing booth, then, towel-loined, to a cabinet inside which she seats him, clamping its door shut around his neck. Steam swirls around his enclosed limbs and torso, making them wet and dry at the same time, immersing him without immersing him *in* anything. Drops form on his forehead and run down his face. It's sweat and sulphur mixed together: licking it from his lips since he can't use his constrained hands to wipe it off, Serge tastes the bitter sootiness again. He spends what seems like hours inside the cabinet. When he's finally released he sees that the sweat that's poured from him is dirty, a blue-black, as though he were full of ink.

He's sent through to an adjoining room to be massaged. The nurse who performs this is only two or three years older than him, short and dark-haired. Her hands make circular passes around his navel, the ball of the hand pressing down into his abdomen before descending in spiralling ovals towards his pelvis; then they move up and down his sides, slapping and sawing. Her body, as she bends above him, seems a funny shape. Her skin is ruddy; her arms and body give off the same musty, sulphurous smell that pervades the corridors, as though her flesh had imbibed it and turned each of her pores into mini-fountains. When she finishes the massage and straightens up, Serge realizes that the unusual shape of her body wasn't just due to her position as she bent, stroking and kneading, over him: her back is slightly crooked.

'Finish now. Same again tomorrow,' she says. Her voice is low and earthy. She has a glazed look, not quite in the present, as though she were staring through him, or around him, at something that was there before he came and will be there after he leaves.

Serge is meant to have a class with Clair after lunch, but he's too exhausted. He sleeps till almost four, then makes his way over to Dr Filip's. In the waiting room, he finds the other patients resting their sample-filled jars across their knees, or on the seat beside them. His is waiting for him in Dr Filip's office: the doctor's holding it up, turning it around and inspecting it when he walks in.

'Not good; very much not good,' Dr Filip says disapprovingly. 'Please to look.'

He hands the jar to Serge. On its outside is a label bearing the handwriting of the nurse who hydro-mined him for its contents. The matter inside is solid, liquorice black, with an undulating surface in whose folds and creases small reserves of dark red moisture have collected.

'Blood,' says Dr Filip, pointing. 'You have cachectic condition: encumbrances in bowel causing autointoxication. Ptomaines, toxins, pathogens all enter bloodstream. Look how dark it is.'

'You mean the blood?' Serge asks. 'Or ...'

'Both,' snaps Dr Filip. 'And if not treated, more. You have a poison factory in you that secretes to arteries, liver, kidneys and beyond. To brain too, when we don't prevent.'

'What's causing it?' Serge asks.

'Morbid matter!' Dr Filip's thin voice pipes from his small mouth. 'Bad stuff. If I am speaking several hundred years ago I call it *chole*, bile – black bile: *mela chole*. Now, I can call it epigastritis, alimentary toxaemia, intestinal putrefaction, or six or seven other names – but these do not explain what causes it. It needs a host to nurture it, and you are willing. Yesterday you spoke to me of what it wants, which means you serve its needs, make them your own. This we must change.'

'How?' Serge asks.

Dr Filip's whiskers rustle as his lips curl in a wry smile. 'I cannot tell you this,' he says. 'You must discover. I can prescribe treatment and diet, monitor symptoms. The rest is for you.' He slips a sheet of paper from his drawer and starts to write. 'Take this to chemist,' he tells Serge. 'The pills, one time each day – not more: too many all at once will kill you. And drink the water, always, all day long. If abdomen distends a little, not to worry. Like your own Lord poet Tennyson has said of faith: "Let it grow."' His eyes glow slightly, like thin filaments, registering satisfaction at the quip he's just made. Then their grey-metallic colour returns as he tells Serge: 'Please to go now.'

III

Serge settles into a routine. Each morning he wanders through the park and sips from the Mir fountain to the sound of orchestra music, then heads on to Letna for a water-and-paraffin-oil enema, then to his hydrotherapy and massage session with the musty-smelling, crook-backed nurse. The lightening effect produced by the enema stays with him through the massage and on until just after lunch, when the veil thickens again and he sleeps for an hour. In the afternoons he has his lessons and takes walks around the town. He dines with Clair each evening, then spends an hour or so reading or playing games in the parlour: dominoes or bridge if in a group of four or five, or, if alone with Clair, chess. In his room, he drinks the bottles that are left for him every morning, with the heart-and-cherub logo and the patent number on their labels; each night he falls asleep with sulphur and soot on his tongue.

Serge gets to know the other patients staying in the hotel. They're always kind to him: as the youngest one, he's treated like a type of mascot. Besides Herr Landmesser and the Dutch woman, Tuithof, there's a Frenchman, Monsieur Bulteau, who takes pleasure in explaining how each person's diet acts on their metabolism, trotting out the names of chemicals, compounds and gastric juices; a Russian, Pan Suchyx, who reads sheet music in a deep armchair each evening, humming the odd snatch out to himself as though pondering a proposition or a line of argument; an Austrian banker named Kleinholz who keeps whipping from his waistcoat pocket a notebook full of columns of what Serge assumes to be ledgers or accounts, and annotating these with a pen he keeps attached to it; and a score of vague Hungarians, Swedes, Serbs and Italians who nod and smile at Serge each time they pass him beside the stuffed animals or on the staircase.

Monsieur Bulteau has a theory about the cysteine, which he expounds one morning in the drawing room.

'For gunpowder, *n'est-ce pas*? Explosion: *pow*!' His hands fly apart in an explosive gesture. 'The Prussians take it to their *arsenales*, prepare for war.'

'*Ganz lächerlich*!' a German lady mutters as she sips her coffee.

Kleinholz, notebook out, starts annotating figures with more rigour. Herr Landmesser declares: 'The earth belongs to Prussia from long time ago, so she may use it as she wishes.'

'How does it belong to Prussia?' Clair asks.

'The whole region is Germanic, from way back,' Herr Landmesser explains. 'This Jiři in the statue, patron saint, is just new, Christian name for old Germanic god.'

'What god would that be?' a Hungarian demands.

'Jirud. He was a prince expulsed from kingdom after he became diseased, and wandered as a swineherd. When he saw his pigs rolling in earth here, and their diseases ended, he did same and was himself cured. Then founded new kingdom here, and conquered back old one too. He was father of Volsung, who is father of Sigmund, father of Sigurd.'

'But,' says Serge, 'no one knew about the healing powers of Kloděbrady until Baron von Arnow found the water under the castle and Maxbrenner plumbed it through the town.'

'You have eaten modern version of story like a good boy taking medicine,' Herr Landmesser informs him with a patronizing glance.

'This is Prussian arrogance *typique*!' Monsieur Bulteau almost shouts, his hands still gunpowdering apart. 'They think all Europe's theirs, and make these stupid *mythes* to justify their avarice for land and power.'

'*Mossieu!*' The German lady slams her coffee down, red-faced. 'You are not polite.'

'She's right: you should apologize,' Herr Landmesser tells Monsieur Bulteau.

'I shall not!' Monsieur Bulteau answers.

The argument rumbles on throughout the day. It spreads to Dr Filip's waiting room, their voices drawing him out of his office to sternly tell all parties to desist.

'Same problem in their heads as in your body,' he tuts as he prods Serge's abdomen back in his office, ear lowered as it tunes into his intestines again. 'Blood of Europe poisoned and cachectic; ptomaines and pathogens in system. Now the black bile is everywhere: the *mela chole*. All have clouded vision, just like you.'

Discussions, hostile or otherwise, become less common as the hotel's population dwindles in late August. Each day the porters' suitcase-laden trolleys clank and trundle down the main drag from the hotel to the station, not the other way. The orchestra by the Mir fountain reduces its appearances to two a week, and even then is made up of fewer musicians than before, its heart shape retained but shrunk, the music now competing with the sound of workmen's hammers banging at stone and plaster as they renovate the mausoleums. Sections of the fountain complex are switched off, drained and repaired. Serge spends whole mornings following the piping's layout, fascinated by the bare mechanics of it all: the joins and junctions where the network splits, the small electric pumps beside the pipes, the insulated wires threaded through these. The habit catches: he starts looking at the ground all day whatever part of town he's in, inspecting the cracks that run through it like skeins, its dark and viscous coloration, or the discarded stubs of bath season tickets and medicine labels ground into it and broken down until they seem as old and organic as earth itself.

IV

At the beginning of September, an arrival creates a small eddy in the flow of leavers from the town. She turns up in the Grand Hotel's lobby with a large round hatbox, a mink stole, a folded parasol of the same light blue as the hatbox, a black handbag and a flotilla of smaller bags and boxes. As porters duck and tack around her, she stands static as a lighthouse in a busy harbour, leaving her older chaperone to issue instructions and distribute tips.

Serge is heading out of the hotel towards the Mir, and half stops when he sees her. She's about his age – perhaps a year or two older, like the crook-backed nurse. She looks at him quizzically when his passage through the lobby falters, which makes him look back quizzically at her, as though he knew her, or perhaps were supposed to perform some task for her that's slipped his mind. She seems to understand the situation sooner than he does – to understand there *is* no situation – and releases his gaze with a confident, if mannered, kind of smile.

He sees her next that afternoon, in the town's museum. The museum's in the castle; Serge didn't even know of its existence until Mevrou Tuithof gushed about it over dinner last night. When he buys a half-crown ticket at its entrance, the old lady in the ticket booth comes round to his side of the window and leads him towards an ancient gramophone in the main gallery.

'*Deutsch*? *Französisch*?' she asks, smiling up at him.

'English,' he replies.

'Ah!' She seems a little shocked, and scurries back to her booth, returning with a record that she lowers to the turntable with shaky hands. Stooping slightly, she leads the pickup's arm across, then down. She turns to Serge now, and makes to say something – but, lacking the English words to do so, merely points to her ear: *listen*. Serge listens. A deep, male, English voice comes crackling through the speaking horn:

'Of all the towns in Central Europe,' it informs him, 'few have had a history so steeped in violence as Kloděbrady.' As though to illustrate its point, a scream – perhaps a child's, perhaps a woman's – interrupts the monologue. 'Here it was,' the deep, male voice continues after the scream fades out, 'that the child-prince of Kutna Hora was beheaded at the order of the *Hauptmann* of Olbec; here it was that Vincenzo and Rosnata, the sons of Mstislav, were killed by Vladimir after their own father's demise.'

Serge nods at the old lady knowingly.

'The *tumour*-humour thing,' he says.

She smiles back at him anxiously, then beats a slow retreat towards her booth. The deep, male voice continues telling him of wars and purges, plagues and fires. He looks around the gallery: its vitrines, made from the same murky glass as the pike-and-otter cases in the hotel, hold illuminated manuscripts depicting scenes of battle and execution. Larger images of similar events hang on the walls. A tapestry of roughly the same size as the one above the staircase at Versoie shows some kind of torture taking place: an unhappy-looking character is being carried by two soldiers up a ladder leading to the rim of a huge vat from which steam rises, while a courtier type points to the vat malevolently. Serge wanders over and inspects the scene more closely. The courtier has the same sharp, narrow features as Dr Filip. Maybe Dr Filip's just the latest incarnation of a character as old as this town itself, Serge thinks to himself – a figure who reappears in era after era. The borders of the tapestry are embellished with insects. Serge turns away from it and feels his veiled vision darkening further, and feels too the dark matter in his stomach tightening, solidifying. The deep voice on the gramophone is talking about the region's landscape.

'... already crossed by an extremely important long-distance trading route linking the centre of the country to the Kodsko region and Silesia inking the centre of the country to the Kodsko region and Silesia inking the centre of the country to the Kod ...'

The record's stuck. Serge turns and makes to walk back to the gramophone so he can release the needle, but sees that he's been beaten to it: a woman, not the ticket lady, is lifting the arm up and sliding it above the record's surface before lowering it back again, allowing the monologue to advance.

'... for the transportation of the mineral-rich earth of the surrounding countryside, which remains a valuable resource to this day. At the beginning of the thirteenth century ...'

The woman turns round now, and he sees it's the new arrival. She's changed since this morning, and now wears an emerald-green knotted cloche hat and a sea-blue shawl.

'My stumbling porter,' she says. 'What's your name?'

He tells her.

'Serge like "sedge", or "urge"?' she asks.

'Just like I said it,' he replies. 'What are you called?'

'Lucia,' she answers. 'It's Italian.'

'You don't sound Italian,' he tells her.

'It's my mother,' says Lucia. 'She's from Genoa. My father's English. "Serge" sounds French.'

'It is. My mother also: her family.'

'You have brothers and sisters?'

'No,' he says. 'I had a sister, but not any more.' Then: 'What are you here for?'

'Here? To see the museum,' she says.

'No, I mean here in Kloděbrady.'

'Oh, anaemia,' she tells him, rolling her eyes up like a naughty schoolgirl. 'My blood's too light or something. How about you?'

'The opposite: too dark.'

Lucia giggles. 'How perfect. Shall we visit the gallery?'

They walk through the large hall beneath tapestries and past illuminations, while the gramophone's account of wars, infanticide, betrayal and sedition echoes at them from the room's high walls. The words soften and run together as they step into the cellar, in which rotting boat fragments, the charcoaled skeletons of old canoes, are laid out among sepulchres whose stone reliefs level accounts between aggressors and their victims by giving the faces of both the same worn-down, characterless quality. When they come up to the main gallery again, the voice is telling them how Mstislav tried to buck the murderous local trend by developing and implementing pacifist strategies.

'He was the one with radical oppinions,' says Serge. 'I read about this earlier. He lay the groundwork for Prince Jiři to … Listen …'

'… for the reign of Prince Jiři,' the deep voice says as though completing, or rephrasing, Serge's sentence, 'who submitted to the royal courts of Europe, under the title of *The General Peaceful Organizations*, a blueprint for universal peace.'

'Well, well,' Lucia says, nodding at him wide-eyed and amused. 'Impressive.'

The record's ended now; the gramophone's speaking horn hisses. Outside, they head beneath an arch, only this time it's held up not by cherubs but on strands which protrude from its underside like fleshy tentacles, giving it an octopus- or jellyfish-like look. They pass out of the courtyard towards the town's river, where, beside a boathouse, rowers are lowering their not-yet-charcoaled canoes from a jetty while swimmers in trunks and bathing caps splash friends in paddle boats. A bridge crosses this; Serge and Lucia walk to its middle, then pause and, leaning on the rail, look down over a large double-decker pleasure boat that's waiting for a lock to open.

'How did your sister die?' Lucia asks. They haven't spoken for a while: just walked and watched the river.

Looking at the swirls emerging from beneath the boat's hull, Serge replies: 'She drowned.'

The lock door opens; bubbles rise up from the churning water; the pleasure boat moves on; so do Lucia and Serge. After a few more yards the bridge turns into a weir. Sluice gates beneath it channel and filter the water; above it, at intervals, gatehouses rise like watchtowers. Beyond these, a generating station runs from the weir to the solid ground on the river's far side. Through its mesh windows, Serge can see turbines grinding and whirring, their wheels and belts resembling the strange machine in Dr Filip's office. The building's electric moan hangs in the air and merges with another hum that comes from somewhere else – from higher, growing in volume and aggression like the buzz of a malignant insect. Serge looks up and sees an airplane flying low above the river. Lucia grabs his shoulder as it passes over them.

'Look!' she shouts, all excited. 'Look at that!'

'It's taking people on an aerial tour of the town and countryside,' Serge says. 'They do it two or so times each week, when the weather's good.'

'Have you flown on it?' she asks.

'No.' Clair suggested it one day but he declined, for the simple reason that he didn't believe that all his weight could possibly get airborne. He knew it could, of course, knew that the laws of physics would allow the machine to bear him on its wings and propeller up into the sky – but *psychologically* ... In his mind the morbid matter Dr Filip spoke of has taken on proportions far, far larger than his stomach could ever accommodate, and expanded to become a landscape, a whole territory: the land itself, and then the murky, gauzy air above it, the dark waters flowing beneath this ... How could all *that* be elevated? His abdomen's swollen since he arrived here. Dr Filip said that this was good – that it was the pure, air-filled water that was swelling it, that purity, like faith, would grow. But something else is growing inside Serge. He feels its heaviness. He sees its heaviness everywhere: in the scales hanging above the doors of chemists' shops, the snakes that curl around them, weighing them down, in the cysteine-rich ballast being crane-hoisted on to groaning trains, or in the hearts that jets and cherubs strain to hold up against dragging weeds and tentacles. He's taken to colouring the hearts black in idle moments in his room: on the stationery beside his bed or on the labels of the mineral-water bottles ...

He sees Lucia often. They take walks together on most afternoons. Both Clair and Lucia's chaperone, the fifty-odd-year-old Miss Larkham, seem to think their company is good for one another. Lucia likes his, certainly: each time she laughs she fixes his eyes with hers, aquamarine and pale, holding them for longer each time. After a few days she starts punching him lightly on the arm whenever she makes a light-hearted comment, or grabbing his shoulder like she did when the airplane flew overhead and leaving her hand there, letting him support her as though she were about to lose her balance even though the patch of ground they're on is straight and flat. He senses that she'd let him return the gesture if he felt like it, and hold her as closely or tightly as he liked, kiss her, do whatever he pleased.

But he's not sure that he wants to. For all Lucia's levity and brightness, he prefers the company of his crook-backed masseuse. Her name's Tania, he found out the third or fourth time she massaged him. He likes the way her hands circle around his stomach, the aggression of the palm's ball pressing down into his flesh and muscles, the spiralling descent that follows, then the way she slaps and saws his sides. He likes her ruddy skin and musty, sulphurous odour; as she bends above him he inhales it deeply, as though breathing in, through her, the sulphurous fumes gushing straight from the springs. Walks with Lucia are enjoyable and pass the time, but sessions with Tania fill him with anticipation, so much so that he finds himself growing impatient for the next morning's one each afternoon, losing the signal of whatever Lucia's talking to him about as his mind tunes forwards to the mustiness, the pressing and descent …

'You turn over now,' she tells him.

As he turns, her distended shoulder looms above him. He likes her crippled body, the illness inside it. Like her smell, it seems to convey something else – something gurgling upwards from below, running through her as though she were a conduit, a set of pipes. Her glazed look too: the way her eyes seem almost oblivious to what's in front of them, fixing instead on something other than the immediate field of vision, deeper and more perennial …

Does his health improve? Not really. Its progress certainly isn't to the satisfaction of the old judge and torturer. He sees Dr Filip once a week and, lying on his back while the detector-whiskers twitch and bristle and the tapper-arm hovers above his abdomen, is lectured on his failings as a patient.

'So: appears your body is responding to the treatment only so it then can reintoxify,' the doctor's sharp voice scolds.

'What's reintoxifying it?' Serge asks.

'*What*? There is no *what*. It reintoxifies itself.'

'*With* what then?' Serge tries.

'Not *with* either. Your illness is not a thing; it is a process. A rhythm. Toxins are secreted around body, organs become accustomed and, perverted by custom, addicted. So when toxins are gone, organs ask for more. More ptomaines, please! More pathogens! And body makes more. The rhythm is repeating, on and on. It will repeat until you – I mean your will, your mind – tell it to stop.'

'How do I tell it that?' Serge asks.

Dr Filip stops tapping; his thin eyes lock on Serge's from behind their steel-rimmed spectacles. 'Tell me,' he says; 'you like it here?'

Serge shrugs. 'It's fine.'

'You like the rhythm of your days? The enemas, the hydrotherapy, the walks …'

'It's rather pleasant,' Serge tells him.

The thin eyes glint metallically. 'See? You find it pleasant – and I think you find the rhythm of your illness pleasant too. It pleases you to feast on the *mela chole*, on the morbid matter, and to feast on it repeatedly, again, again, again, like it was lovely meat – lovely, black, rotten meat. And so the rotten meat pollutes your soul.'

'But if I like it here,' Serge counters, 'and follow what's prescribed, doesn't that mean I'm accepting of the treatment rather than resistant to it?'

Dr Filip turns from him and fiddles with his instruments. His small, tight back seems tense with thinking. After a while he answers: 'Things mutate. That is the way of nature – of good nature: things pass through on their way to somewhere else, and both they and the things they pass through are thereby transformed. You following me?'

'I suppose so,' Serge says hesitantly.

'You, though,' the doctor continues, 'have got blockage. Jam, block, stuck. Instead of transformation, only repetition. Need to free what's blocking, break whole rhythm of intoxication – then good transformation can resume and things will pass through you and make you open up. You still are only adolescent: still have much transformation to perform. Blockage must be broken, then body and soul both will open up, like flowers.'

In mid-September there's a religious festival. Lucia finds it all very amusing. She and Serge shadow the procession as it emerges from the doors of the town's church and makes its way towards the castle, after which it heads down to first the Letna, then the Maxbrenner buildings, pausing to perform a ceremony on the steps of each. It then moves past the rows of chemists' shops and the kiosks lining the main drag, each one of which it blesses too; then, finally, across the lawns of the fountain park, where it takes in all the mausoleums before ending up beside the Mir. At its head a priest, holding aloft a cross, intones liturgical script, while sub-priests and altar boys murmur assent. The orchestra, heart shape abandoned, follow behind, intermittently striking up tunes that sound rather funereal, breaking these off, then striking them up again, reprising the same passages. The townspeople who move along its route with Lucia and Serge join in at regular intervals, reciting short phrases in their own, non-liturgical language.

'What do you think they're saying?' asks Lucia, holding Serge's arm.

'"O holy water, please keep bringing us rich foreigners so that we may take their money,"' Serge answers.

Lucia flings her head back in a peal of laughter and throws both her arms around his neck. A couple of townspeople turn round and cast them disapproving glances. A hush spreads through the crowd as the priest dips his cross into the Mir; then all heads bow as he holds it submerged beneath the water. He keeps it there for a long time. Watching him, Serge is struck by the suspicion that all the water that's gushed through the Mir since its inception would never purify him, wash his dark bile away, because the water's dark as well. It's bubbled up from earth so black that no blessing could ever lighten it, been filtered through the charcoaled wrecks of boats and tumour-ridden bones of murdered ancestors, through stool-archives and other sedimented layers of morbid matter. Serge turns his veiled gaze away from the priest – and as he does, sees Tania looking back at him with old, glazed eyes.

V

By late September only Serge and Clair, Lucia and Miss Larkham and a gaggle of full-time patients who've resigned themselves to the knowledge that they'll never leave the place alive remain in the Grand Hotel. The poles outside stand flagless; the terrace, cleared of tables, collects leaves. The concierge and maître d', as often as not out of uniform, chat to one another across the reception desk even when guests are waiting.

The general relaxation of formalities makes itself felt in Serge's sessions with Tania. There's nothing tangible that's changed: she still wears the same coat and presses, slaps and saws in the same places – but her hands move over him more casually now. Each session seems like a weekend one, as though they'd both just popped into an empty office before slipping off on an excursion. One morning, Serge asks her what she's doing later; when she answers 'I do nothing', he suggests they take a boat ride together.

'Pleasure boat finished now,' she answers. 'Not tourists enough.'

'Well then, we'll hire a paddle boat,' Serge answers. 'Want to come?'

Without pausing her rubbing, she replies: 'What time?'

'Six o'clock,' Serge says. 'Make that five. It's getting dark earlier and earlier these days.'

The boathouse by the lock turns out to be closed. He wonders what to do with Tania while he waits for her in front of it. He waits until five thirty, then five forty-five, then six.

The next day, as she massages him, he asks her why she didn't show up. 'Boathouse closed,' she says. 'Other nurse tell me.'

'Well, we could have gone for a walk,' Serge says.

'Where?' she asks.

'In the woods, for example. They look nice. Why don't we do that this evening?'

'Six o'clock again?' she asks. 'Turn over now.'

'Five,' he says as her shoulder looms above him. 'On the far side of the weir, by the power station.'

'Power?' she asks, sawing his back.

'Yes. You know: electricity.' He makes a moaning noise and wheels his arms around beside his waist.

'I understand,' she says, pushing them down again. 'I come.'

As he waits by the substation he watches soldiers practising manoeuvres in the fields. They run a few feet forwards and lie down, pointing their dummy rifles at the wood, then jump up and run a few feet further before throwing themselves at the earth again, advancing in stops and starts towards some imaginary enemy within the trees. He longs for Tania's musty smell, turns back towards the weir to look for her, and sees that a door in the generating station is opening. A man walks out and says something to him.

'I'm sorry …' Serge shrugs.

'*Deutsch*?'

'No: English.'

'Oh! You English!' The man's face lights up. He's fiftyish, well built, with thick grey hair and bronzed, sinewy arms that look like the vines in the patch he's just stepped out into. 'English good people!'

'Thank you,' Serge says to him. 'Are these vines yours?'

'Vine? Kystenvine, special of region. You like vine?'

'They look nice,' Serge answers.

'I get for you,' the man says, then turns and heads back to the generating station. He emerges a few moments later with a bottle. 'Here: *Geschenk* for good English!' he says, pushing it through the mesh with his strong, wood-dark arm. 'Electro-vine. You take!'

The bottle is made from the same murky glass as everything else around here. Its contents are so dark that at first Serge thinks the man has handed him some bottled local earth; but when he takes it through the fence he realizes there's liquid in it. As he turns it in his hands the liquid runs inside, its silky, deep-red filaments stirring and catching the light until they seem to glow.

'It's wine?' he asks the man. 'From these vines?'

'*Da – ja* – how say? Yes! Kystenvine: we make here, only few bottles, for us. Electro-vine for good electro-men!'

He lets out a deep, hearty laugh, then disappears into the generating station once more. Serge thinks of taking the wine to the field's edge and drinking it as he watches the soldiers train, but realizes that he doesn't have a corkscrew. Returning to the hotel, he slips the bottle beneath his shirt so Clair won't see it.

In his room, a letter's waiting for him. It's from his father.

> Dear Son,
>
> I trust the water's to your liking. As you'll doubtless be aware (or perhaps not, bathed as you are in splendid isolation), the Pontic seas of politics are flowing with compulsive course to the Propontic and the Hellesport. Should a retiring ebb not be felt soon, I fear we'll have to curtail your stay among the Nix and bring you home, lest *Vernichtung* lay down a barrier preventing your return. Await instructions.

Serge sets the letter down. He had a fluoroscopy session one day, quite early in his stay in Kloděbrady, when Dr Filip wanted to ascertain the extent of the encumbrance in his bowels. In a windowless room buried deep in the entrails of the Maxbrenner building, he stood between a lead-lined X-ray box and an empty wooden frame that Dr Filip shifted slightly up and down on its supporting post until it was positioned just in front of Serge's midriff. The doctor then slid a screen into the frame's groove and, stepping away from Serge, switched the room's lights off and the contraption on. There was a whirring, then a flash, a smell of calcium tungstate; and then a glowing pool collected in the air just on the far side of the screen, as though Serge's stomach were seeping light.

'Please not to move,' the doctor's voice instructed him from the darkness as Serge tried to crane his head forwards to see the light source. 'I can show you with mirror.'

A scraping came from beneath the voice, then the sound of something being lifted from the floor – then there it was, reflected back at him: the inside of his belly, etched in blocks and lines of black against the fluoroscope screen's sickly calcium white, suspended in a void that detached it from anything and everything. Organs, tubes and bones quivered and oscillated against each other awkwardly, like animals – reptiles, molluscs, nether-dwelling creatures – who, crammed together in a space too small for them, bristle with aggression towards one another. Both Serge and Dr Filip watched the scene in silence for quite some time. Serge's stomach, and not the vacuum in which it was held, was the living, moving part of this new film that was being projected and viewed in the instant of its creation – and yet, rendered negative and ghostly by the rays, it seemed to Serge more dead than all the meat inside it.

'Why didn't you turn up this time?' he asks as Tania presses her balled palms into his abdomen the next morning.

'I have thing to do,' she answers.

'I met a man who gave me wine,' he tells her.

'Cystenwine?' she asks him.

'That's what he called it, more or less.'

'Is very good.'

'We could drink it together,' he says, 'if you come this evening.'

'OK,' she says, 'I come.'

To his surprise, she does. They meet on the weir and stroll over to the far bank, past the generating station. Serge can see figures moving around inside, but can't tell if his vine-limbed benefactor is among them. He and Tania pass the substation and head into the fields. The soldiers are all gone; the whole landscape seems empty – even the train pulled up beside the earth mounds a quarter of a mile or so away has been abandoned, its driver probably drinking with the shovellers and soldiers, the bandstand painters and dining-hall decorators in one of the town's inns. Serge has the Kystenwein on him; he also has a corkscrew borrowed from the hotel's kitchen. He looks at Tania, wondering if he should break the bottle out right now. She doesn't seem impatient for it. Her eyes, dimmer than usual in the dusk, stare vaguely ahead, towards the woods. A path leads into these; they follow it. After a while the woods end temporarily and a strip, too narrow for a field, runs between them and the next block of woods.

'Against fire,' Tania tells him – the first words she's spoken since they started walking.

'What's one disaster more or less, in this town?' Serge murmurs.

She doesn't respond. To their right, in the firebreak's middle, there's an indentation: a kind of mini-quarry where the ground's been hollowed out. Its black-soiled surfaces curve in a way suggestive of soft chairs.

'Why don't we sit there?' Serge asks.

Tania shrugs. They enter the indentation and sit down, leaning back against its edges. Serge pulls the corkscrew from his pocket and opens the bottle.

'I didn't bring any glasses, I'm afraid,' he tells her.

Tania takes the bottle from his hands and drinks from it, throwing her head back. The liquid casts a deep red glow across her neck. She hands it back to him. He brings it to his lips – and tastes on its rim the warm, bitter residue of Tania's spit. The wine itself he doesn't taste till further back, down in his throat: it's bitter too, in a rich, dirty way.

'It's different from the one I had on my first evening here,' he says. 'My tutor said that it was good for my digestion, but Dr Filip's only letting me drink –'

'Why you come alone with teacher?' Tania interrupts him. 'Why not parents too?'

'They have things to do, like you.'

'Take care of brothers and sisters?'

'No,' Serge replies. 'I don't have those. I had a sister, but no more.'

'She died?' asks Tania. Serge nods. 'How?'

Serge ponders the question for a while, then answers: 'She fell from a height and hit the ground.'

Tania reaches for the bottle and drinks again. When she's done, he drinks too. The wine's making him warm; he feels the silky hotness moving outwards from his stomach, to his arms, his legs, his head. Tania takes the bottle again and drinks once more, this time taking long, deep gulps. He does the same. Some of the wine's escaped from the side of Tania's mouth; it runs down her chin and dribbles on to her blouse. Serge reaches out his hand and spreads the wet film from her chin around her cheek. She doesn't stop him, or react in any way. Her eyes, glazed as always, stare through him at the black earth. He brings his mouth up to her face and licks the wine from it. Her neck, beside his ear, emits a low, guttural sound, of the same character and pitch as low-frequency radio waves. He can smell the musty odour rising from her body – from its corners, enclaves, holes. He tugs at her blouse and, meeting no resistance, pulls it off completely, then does the same to her skirt and underclothes.

'Turn round,' he says. 'I want to see your back.'

She turns. There it is, right under his face: the crook, rising beneath her shoulder like a ridge with valleys running down its side, flesh-rills held up by bones under the skin. He touches it, then runs his fingers up and down the rills. Still kneeling behind her, he pulls his own clothes off and, holding his penis in his right hand, feeds it inside her from behind while clasping her back's crook in his left hand. The guttural sounds in her neck increase in volume; the musty smell grows stronger, sharper. Serge shuts his eyes then opens them again and, looking straight down, sees the earth rising between Tania's fingers where her hands push into it. He runs his own hand down her back, so hard the nails puncture its surface, and moves inside her violently, like he's seen animals and insects do it. Her thighs push back at him, pulling him further in. He closes his eyes again and feels a burning growing in his stomach.

'Poisonberry,' he says, barely audibly.

The word hovers in a small gas cloud of breath over Tania's skin before spreading outwards, dissipating. The burning's spreading outwards too, just like the wine; it's spreading beyond his body, moving out to fill the hollow, and beyond that too, across the firebreak to the woods on either side. A scream, or the echo of a scream, erupts from neither him nor Tania but, it seems, the night itself; and with it comes a tearing sound, as though a fabric were being ripped. Serge opens his eyes now, and finds that the gauzy crêpe that's furred his vision for so long is gone – completely gone, like a burst bubble or disintegrated membrane. The surfaces of ground and woods and clouds are gone too, fallen away like screens, encumbrances that blocked his vision, leaving the hollow – not of the indentation but of space itself: an endless space in which he can now see with piercing clarity. What he sees is darkness, but he sees – sees it. ■

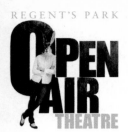

MY QUEER WAR

James Lord

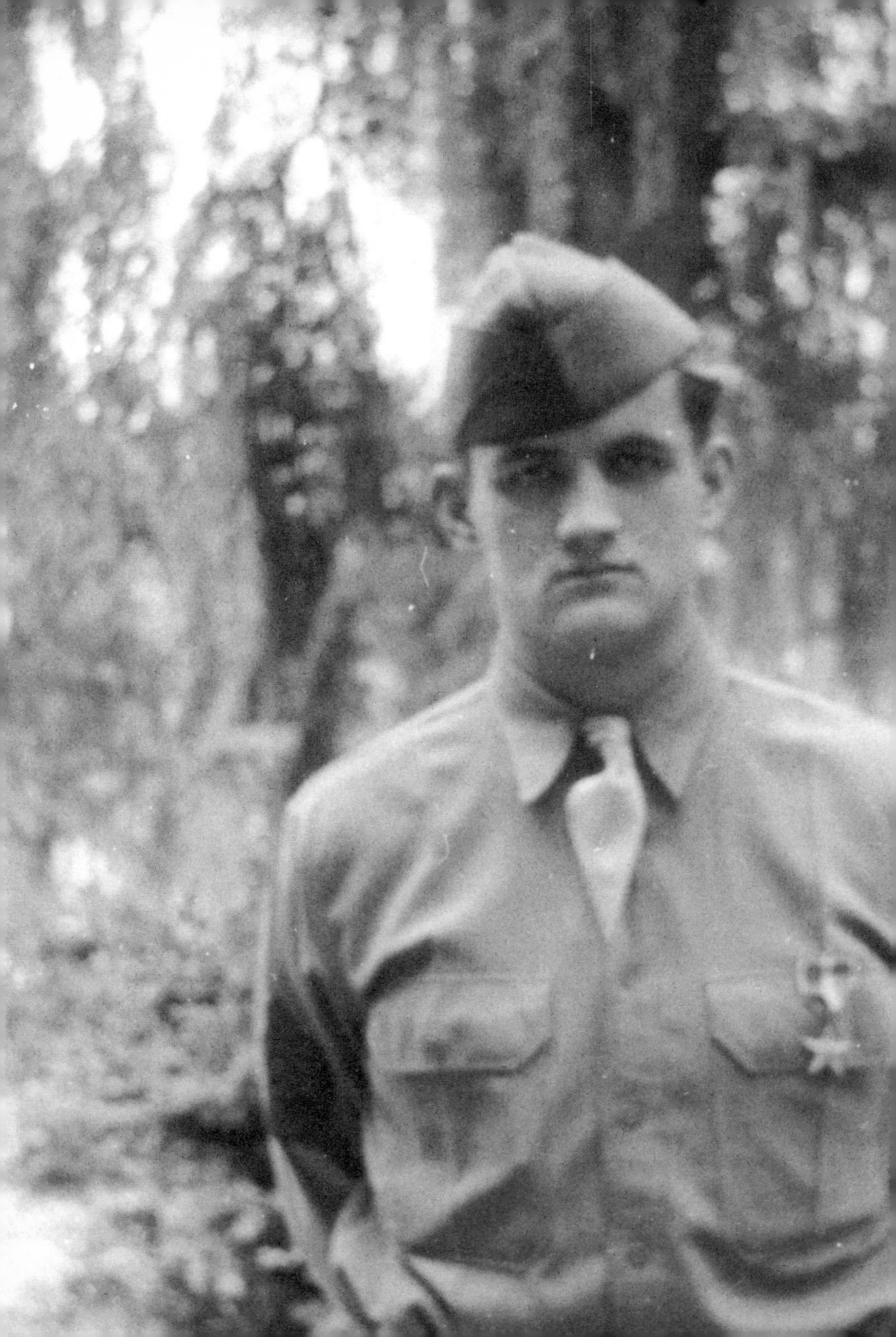

Indian summer was a little late that year, bringing lambent afternoons, miniature whirlwinds of withering leaves, misty sunsets, wild evenings. To one side of the campus lay a strip of lawn secluded behind rhododendron hedges where I liked to linger in the amethyst twilight, a select hideaway for meetings with myself. Then one evening an awareness that I was not alone stole across the grass: a figure in uniform, someone I knew by way of hello only, a PFC from down the hall named Jerry Weinbaum, not in any of our study groups, a guy who laughed a lot, tall, not bad-looking. He said, 'Hi there. Be dark in a few minutes. Mind if I walk along?'

'Course not. How you doing?'

'I make out. You?'

'Oh, sure. Everything's OK.'

'Find Boston friendly then, do you?'

'I do, yes. Nice people. Make you feel right at home.'

'Already found yourself a friend then?'

'One of my room-mates, yes. Comes from Boston. His mother invited me to lunch last Sunday, played the harp; it was beautiful.'

'Say, that must have been all right. Nice lady, huh? Don't hang out with the boys, though, do the bars, drinking, you know, hail-fellow-well-met thing?'

'Not really. I'm not too keen on the USO type, tell the truth.'

'No kidding. Who is? That's not what I meant. I meant making out with guys you really get along with, you know, guys like us.'

I hesitated, not knowing where such desultory talk could go – besides, it was getting dark – not giving a damn, pointless to chat with someone with whom I had nothing in common.

He said, 'Do you mind if I ask you a question?'

'Not at all. Shoot.'

'Are you gay?'

'Funny thing,' I said. 'That lady I mentioned, she said I was a gay blade. She meant somebody without a care in the world, I guess.'

'Come on' – he cut in brusquely – 'that's not what I'm talking about. I spotted you from the beginning. Takes one to know one. So fess up. I'm not the police. Wouldn't come on to you if I wasn't gay myself. Relax.'

He put his hand on my shoulder while I was numbed by surprise and moved his fingertips gently to the nape of my neck, tickling my hair till I shivered and my legs were like danger in deep water.

'You like to make love to boys, don't you?' he said, and when in the trembling silence I didn't say no, he added, 'Do you mind if I kiss you?' and when I didn't say no, he did.

And I kissed him back, letting go of time, place, myself, the swelling seizure of sensation, surrender, sudden nothingness of everything else, no longer knowing what or where or why, and his hands were all over me, fumbling with my clothes, nor did I understand how we were lying on the cool grass in the abrupt dark, so I mumbled, 'But somebody might see us,' in an ecstasy of fear.

'This is your first time, isn't it?' he said in my ear. 'I can tell. I'll show you what it's like. You'll like it. Just let yourself go, baby.'

So I did, and he did, and I did.

The ascent into oblivion was utter caesura of self. I choked against the lament of pleasure, the shock of life, as if I'd waited for it for ever; neither vile nor frightening, it bit me exactly where – and how – the heartbeat of sensation, thoughtless and pure, drove my blood, the freedom of it intoxicating. So this was what it was all about. Yes. And I thought, 'If only.'

But there I was with Jerry in the confusion of our bodies in the grass, now pitch dark, and our clothes were a mess.

He said, 'So you don't know what it means to be gay?'

'Apparently not.'

'It's a password. We use it between ourselves so other people won't know we're talking about being queer. You don't know a thing about the gay scene, do you?'

'I guess I don't.'

'How old are you?'

'Twenty.'

'Late starter. High time you got to know the world you're going to spend your life in. I can give you a shove in that direction if you want. Don't get me wrong, but you've got a lot to learn. I go into Boston weekends. Can show you around. You'll be surprised. I can give you the shove. You sink or swim, that's your business. OK?'

'I guess,' I said.

'Friday then. See you at the bus stop six thirty, forty-five. Button up your pants, sweetheart.'

Was what had happened apparent to my room-mates? Aaron? Tony? They naturally knew that homosexuality was a quotient of the human equation, Oscar Wilde having taken good care to publicize the facts. Jerry considered me innocent; I could play that part for my friends breezily. When Aaron enquired about the weekend, I said I was going to cruise around town on my own, never in my jejune insouciance fancying that that described exactly what I'd do.

Jerry led me along past the Public Garden to the Hotel Statler, telling me never to forget how to get there, as this would be my jumping-off place in Boston.

The lobby was long and high, expensive, gold-plated, busy with wartime visitors. This was where guests registered for the weekend. It paid off to reserve a room in advance, Jerry said, because when cruising the bar, you'd want someplace to do it if you picked up a trick.

The crescent-shaped bar was packed with servicemen, several rows deep, too many to count, a hundred, maybe a hundred and fifty, most of them drinking beer from the bottle, loud with flighty talk and piercing laughter. Crowded tight together, jostling back and forth, not one lady or girl among them, only a handful of civilians.

'Yes,' said Jerry, 'they're all gay.'

'But this is a public place. People who don't know could come in, couldn't they?'

'Oh, yeah. Straights stray in. It happens. But usually they notice something and stray right out again. I mean, we have a right to

Lebensraum, haven't we? Anyway, there's a straight seating area right up there to keep things looking honest.'

Back a polite distance from the bar, up three or four steps behind a metal grille, were a lot of small tables, clients seated there, a proviso of women among them, waiters in snappy jackets dancing around to serve them.

'But don't they know?' I wondered. 'Can't they tell?'

'Hell, no. Decent people don't want to know. And anyway, they couldn't tell if their grandmothers sold snuggle on the side. It's an obstacle course getting to the bar to get served. Use your elbows. But watch out for your pants. It can get real feely in this crowd.'

Elbows, knees and 'sorry' got us through. Jerry asked for a Rheingold. I said Tom Collins.

Some of the servicemen were exciting to look at, and some of them obviously knew it, glancing round the crowd with chancy eyes and the aura pervasive throughout was edgy-sexy readiness for anything. I'd never known the like or known myself like an element of it.

An English marine lance corporal in dress uniform wedged along in front of me, said, 'Hi there, Yankee Doodle, what say we make out below stairs in the Gents?' his fingers fooling free-and-easy with the buttons of my fly.

Of course in the confines of the crowd it would have been difficult to see what he was doing, and he was good-looking enough, ruddy, bright-eyed, brawny in the tight-fitting uniform; and the incursion of his fingers roused me all right, though his breath in my face was brewery, and I knew perfectly well what the Gents meant; it was shocking that I wasn't all that shocked, yet I couldn't let myself go so easily so soon, and I brushed aside his hand, saying – but with a gasp – 'Sorry. Some other time.'

Jerry was chatting up a lieutenant in pinks – yes, there were a few officers – but I bumped between and said, 'Can't we get out of here? I need some air.'

'Christ,' Jerry gurgled. 'Hold on, will you? Let me say a word to Glen for a minute. I'll catch up with you in the lobby.'

We walked up Tremont opposite the Common, to Schrafft's, and had some pot roast and blueberry pie. Jerry told me I'd better settle down and learn what I wanted to do about what was inside my pants or I might turn out to be one sad and lonely faggot. It was common sense speaking, I knew, but I felt the gnaw of worry I'd be found wanting when called to act on the lesson of my sexual ABCs.

'Back to the Statler?' I asked when we came out on to the sidewalk.

'Better try something else,' said Jerry. 'Now you know your way to the Statler you can touch base there any time. Now's a good time for the Napoleon.'

'Napoleon? As in Bonaparte? You must be kidding.'

'Hell, no. Shit, ever since Alex the Great and his boyfriend what's-his-name, groovy guys in uniform are doable, and anyway, Alex didn't go in much for clothes, did he? The Napoleon's a gay club. Right down here.'

In the darkling side street, the houses all looked stunted, their doors steeped in secrets, to which our presence brought no enlightenment, and I wondered how the hell I was going to get out of this.

He pressed a button, a piercing light lit the doorway, a peephole popped open, and he said, 'Hi there, honey child, it's your uncle Wiggly.'

Honey child was a black six-footer wearing a purple T-shirt and apple-green skullcap. 'Hello, Auntie,' he said. 'You come in. Bring your boyfriend.'

'Just say my friend's friend's all,' said Jerry. 'Trust him in your hands, honey, you give him a push. Me, I've got a date, gonna boogie with a looie at the Ritz.'

Jerry pinched my behind. 'You're on your own, Jim. You'll be OK. See you back at St Mary's.' And he skipped away into the incautious dark.

Honey child led me inside. A staircase with a cherry-red carpet and a pink droplet chandelier. He said, 'You trot upstairs now like a good boy, find yourself any friend, you hear me,' and he gently prodded the small of my back.

In the high, long room upstairs a comfortable crowd of men eddied along the bar; there was a huge painting of Napoleon astride a charger and a baby white upright piano against the other wall, a bald gent in a tuxedo tickling the ivories and singing 'Mad About the Boy' in a whispering falsetto.

'Are you?' someone murmured in my ear.

'What?' I exclaimed, turning. 'What is it?'

'Like that?' said the stranger, a dark-haired, tan-cheeked young fellow in civvies, nodding at the singer, who was still singing about being mad about a boy.

'Are you?' asked my interlocutor again.

The entertainer flung up his hands, turning to face the crowd and gave a seated bow to the sputtering of applause, his face florid with make-up, mascara and rouge, and some of the red had rubbed off onto his teeth so that the show-business smile was a bit Bela Lugosi as Dracula.

'Well,' insisted my neighbour, 'are you?'

Then I looked at him. Tall, slender, in a navy-blue suit, eyes amber with an intense sapphire tint but smiling, friendly, dimpled cheeks. So I said, 'Well, am I?'

'Mad about a boy? Must be, I'd think, hanging out in this place, no?'

I said, 'Must be.'

'Shall we drink to it?'

'Why not?'

He walked to the bar, his gait, it seemed, slightly askew, not quite a limp but not the automatic stride of youth either. It gave him an air, somewhat *distingué*, attractive. Like a diplomat, I thought, on duty at the consulate in Palermo. He ordered Scotch and soda for two.

I said, 'Why is this place called the Napoleon?'

'Why not? All his soldiers were in love with him. Stationed in Boston, are you?'

'Chestnut Hill, Boston College. Special training programme.'

'Cushy. Better off than GI Joe slogging around in the Italian rain.'

'You bet.' I laughed. 'And you? You live here?'

'That's right. Just around the corner, as a matter of fact. I suppose you're wondering, aren't you? People do. I must be the only civilian in here. All these beautiful uniforms, and look at me.'

What I saw was a handsome man about twenty-five years old, wearing a white shirt and a necktie matching his eyes. 'So what?'

'I'm four-F. You may have noticed. The limp. Could call it the FDR exemption. Caught polio as a kid. Lucky, though. Only one leg affected, and not too bad. I can hop, but I can't skip.'

'Well then, you're better off than the president. Lots of jobs in civvy street these days anyway. So you build airplanes or something?'

He smiled and offered me a cigarette. He was in control, as if appraising the terms of a plenipotentiary transaction. 'I'm a sort of architect, pretty good with blueprints, you know. What's your name?'

'Jim,' I said, taken aback by the quick simplicity of his superiority. 'Jim Lord.'

'Nice name. I like it,' he said. 'Jim. Mine's Gordon. Haney. Gordon Haney. You're on your own, are you?'

'Sure,' I said, thinking Jerry would have told me, in any case, I'd better be. 'I'm on my own.'

'Like to come to my place for a drink then?'

I swallowed hard on his invitation, but it was what I was here for, and I cleared my throat to say, 'Yes. Sure. I'd like to.'

Gordon gave me a very accomplished grin, paid for our drinks, and we went to the stairway past the portrait of the soldier beloved by soldiers.

Around the corner turned out to lie several streets distant in the night now too quiet, and Gordon kept time with our steps telling stories of the city's history.

It wasn't too long, or long enough, before we came to his place. It lay down a walled passageway giving on to a courtyard where three trees still held a few faded leaves, and two small brick houses faced each other above an antique lantern. 'Eighteen twenty-six,' said Gordon. 'Built by a whaler for his twin sons, Ebenezer and Jedediah Spooner. We live on the left hand, of course, the Ebenezer House,' as he unlocked the white door.

I followed up three flights to an attic room, narrow and snug with a sloping ceiling, a divan to the right with cushions heaped against the wall, a couple of chairs, a record player, orange lights turned low, and a glass door at the end opening on to a flat roof. He said sit down, make yourself comfortable, take off your jacket and tie, take a deep breath. I'll make us a drink. And he went back downstairs. Undoing the top two buttons of my shirt, I wasn't afraid. I was terrified. Knowing perfectly well why I was there, only wanting to be there. With this stranger, his gazelle-like limp and capable eyes. Would he find me inadequate, clumsy, ignorant, timid, a fool, a mistake? I was ready for anything, prepared for nothing. And what had happened with Jerry would be no good to me now, because now I had to know *myself*, to be something, become someone I didn't know.

Gordon came back, clinking glass in each hand, sat beside me on the divan and said, 'A little music maybe. Rocky Two?'

I swallowed. 'What's that?'

'Rachmaninov. The Second Piano Concerto.'

'OK.'

'Come on, Jim. Don't be nervous.'

I lied, 'I'm not, I'm not nervous.'

'Yes, you are. You are. Here. Look at me.'

He took my face in both of his hands, drawing me to him, to his mouth, kissing, searching with his lips tentatively at first, gently, then more tenaciously as I opened to him, responsive to his mouth in mine, holding on to him to save my life.

He held me back an inch from his face. 'Do you want to take your clothes off by yourself, or would you like me to do it?'

Someone else speaking for me said, 'Yes, please, you do it.'

He did it. Ever so slowly, so tenderly, button by button, easing away shirt, shoes and socks, pants, while at the same time guiding my hands to do the same for him, and he contrived too to turn off the nearby lights so we were in each other's shadow, and it was amazing, as if such gestures and facility had been born and bred in both of us from a time before we knew what we were doing, and we were naked together on the divan among the jumble of cushions, and it was all right, altogether, everything that he did to me, and with me, that I did likewise to him and with him, and I wanted ever so much to be more, far more, and for him, and it was, it was for him and because of him when the crescendo of sensation became complete ... then the silence of our breathing.

Motionless, wordless, we waited. He handed me a glass. I held it against my wet stomach. He lit a cigarette. Then there intruded a sound as of a fluttering of winged things outside, touching the door's glass panes. It was raining.

'That was good,' he said. 'You know, you're very sweet to make love to. Are you all right?'

'Yes,' I said, wanting to whisper to him, 'I'm all right, yes.'

'I'm glad. You can stay over if you like. There are clean sheets and a blanket under the coverlet, a bathroom on the half landing outside. Better to stay over unless you have to be someplace early Sunday.'

He stood up, and I did notice then that his left leg was thinner than the right, though not unsightly. Having put out the cigarette, he gathered up his clothes and shoes in a bundle under one arm, his drink in the other hand, and said pleasant dreams.

In the morning take a shower, shave. Come down any time you're ready. We get up early. Waffles for breakfast on Sundays. And a glass of champagne. Nothing's too good for a member of our armed forces.

We? To be sure, he'd said 'we' at the front door, but I could have assumed he meant the two of us then. And why had he not stayed to sleep beside the body it had been sweet to make love to? I wondered in the sudden solitude, the flutter of raindrops against the glass speechless.

The bathroom was almost overly immaculate, too well appointed to allow you to feel at home, so you supposed you weren't supposed to. I went alone to turn out the lights and go to sleep on the destitute divan.

An abrupt brightness jerked me awake the next day. There was a confusion of blankets, sunlight, but no naked body beside mine, and I suddenly ached for Gordon, anxious again for the desire and the bafflement.

I took a cold shower, shaved, dressed and went downstairs. ■

ZEPPELIN

Herta Müller

TRANSLATED BY PHILIP BOEHM

Behind the factory is a place with no coke ovens, no extractor fans, no steaming pipes, where the tracks come to an end, where all we can see from the mouth of the coal silo is a heap of rubble overgrown with flowering weeds, a pitiful bare patch of earth at the edge of the wilderness, criss-crossed by well-trodden paths. There, out of sight to all but the white cloud drifting far across the steppe from the cooling tower, is a gigantic rusted pipe, a discarded seamless steel tube from before the war. The pipe is seven or eight metres long and two metres high and has been welded together at the end closest to the silo. The end that faces the wilderness is open. A mighty pipe, no one knows how it wound up here. But everyone knows what purpose it has served since we arrived in the camp. It's called the Zeppelin.

This Zeppelin may not float high and silver in the sky, but it does set your mind adrift. It's a by-the-hour hotel tolerated by the camp administration and the bosses, the *nachalniks* – a trysting place where the women from our camp meet with German POWs who are clearing the rubble in the wasteland or in the bombed-out factories. Wildcat weddings was how Anton Kovacs put it: open your eyes sometime when you're shovelling coal, he told me.

As late as the summer of Stalingrad, that last summer on the veranda at home, a love-thirsty female voice had spoken from the radio, her accent straight from the Reich: Every German woman should give the Führer a child. My aunt Fini asked my mother: How are we to do that? Is the Führer planning to come here to Siebenbürgen every night, or are we supposed to line up one by one and visit him in the Reich?

We were eating jugged hare; my mother licked the sauce off a bay leaf, pulling the leaf slowly through her mouth. And when she had licked it clean, she stuck it in her buttonhole. I thought they were only pretending to make fun of him. The twinkle in their eyes suggested they'd be more than a little happy to oblige. My father noticed as well: he wrinkled his forehead and forgot to chew for a while. And my grandmother said: I thought you didn't like men with moustaches. Send the Führer a telegram that he better shave first.

Since the silo yard was vacant after work and the sun still glaring high above the grass, I went down the path to the Zeppelin and looked inside. The front of the pipe was shadowy, the middle was very dim and the back was pitch dark. The next day I opened my eyes while I was shovelling coal. Late in the afternoon I saw three or four men coming through the weeds. They wore quilted work jackets like ours, except theirs had stripes. Just outside the Zeppelin they sat down in the grass up to their necks. Soon a torn pillowcase appeared on a stick outside the pipe – a sign for *occupied*. A while later the little flag was gone. Then it quickly reappeared and disappeared once more. As soon as the first men had gone, the next three or four came and sat down in the grass.

I also saw how the women work brigades covered for each other. While three or four wandered off into the weeds, the others engaged the *nachalnik* in conversation. When he asked about the ones that had stepped away they explained it was because of stomach cramps and diarrhoea. That was true, too, at least for some – but of course he couldn't tell for how many. The *nachalnik* chewed on his lip and listened for a while, but then kept turning his head more and more frequently in the direction of the Zeppelin. At that point I saw how the women had to switch tactics; they whispered to our singer, Loni Mich, who began singing loud enough to shatter glass – drowning out all the noise made by our shovelling:

Evening silence on the vale
Except a lonely nightingale

– and suddenly all the ones who had disappeared were back. They crowded in among us and shovelled away as if nothing had happened.

I liked the name Zeppelin: it resonated with the silvery forgetting of our misery, with the quick, catlike coupling ... I realized that these unknown German men had everything our men were lacking. They had been sent by the Führer into the world as warriors, and they were also the right age, neither childishly young nor overripe like our men were. Of course they, too, were miserable and degraded, but they had seen battle, had fought in the war. For our women they were heroes, a notch above the forced labourers, and offered more than evening love in a barrack bed behind a blanket. The evening love remained indispensable. But for our women it smelled of their own hardship, the same coal and the same longing for home. And it always led to the same give and take. The man provided the food; the woman cleaned and consoled. Love in the Zeppelin was free of every worry except for the hoisting and lowering of the little white flag.

Anton Kovacs was convinced I would disapprove of the women going to the Zeppelin. No one could have guessed that I understood them all too well, that I knew all about arousal in pulled-down pants, about stray desires and gasping delight in the alder park and the Neptune baths. No one could imagine that I was reliving my own trysts, more and more often: Swallow, Fir, Ear, Thread, Oriole, Cap, Hare, Cat, Seagull. Then Pearl. No one had any idea I was carrying so many cover names in my head, and so much silence on my back.

Even inside the Zeppelin, love had its seasons. The wildcat weddings came to end in our second year, first because of the winter and later because of the hunger. When the hunger angel was running rampant during the skin-and-bones time, when male and female could not be distinguished from each other, coal was still unloaded at the silo. But the path in the weeds was overgrown. Purple-tufted vetch clambered among the white yarrow and the red orache, the blue burdocks bloomed and the thistles as well. The Zeppelin slept and belonged to the rust, just like the coal belonged to the camp, the grass belonged to the steppe and we belonged to hunger. ■

POEM | C. K. WILLIAMS

Bianca Burning

The sexual terror lions are roaring into my ears as I make my way between their cages
at the Bertram Mills circus in England in nineteen fifty-seven when I'm twenty.
The terrible lions have roared for six months and though I don't know it they'll roar
for six more then be extinguished, leaving only their irksome echo the rest of my life.

A circus – I'm travelling with a *circus*, an exotic thing to think, and I have a Bianca –
not the Bianca Bruno Schulz had in his 'Spring', an 'enchanting' Bianca whom one
'would notice ... how with every step light as a dancer she enters her being ...' – a Bianca,
rather, who's lush, ardent, and, though only eighteen, more amorously advanced than I am,

with breasts too beautiful to remember and that other thing further down she'll bring
with her every day to my 'digs' to roll with me on my bed, while I flail and despair,
and return with her back through that savage alley, that gauntlet of error and terror,
to the 'caravan' where her father and mother lived, and where we ate dinner together.

Bianca's father is a clown. Not the way I was a clown, a sexual clown, not the way
Schulz depicts himself in his drawings as almost a clown, with his rack of compulsions –
Bianca's father's a real clown, famous, with different names in different countries,
who in the ring in his Chaplinesque costume is hilarious, reckless, contagiously joyful.

Yet Bianca's father like me is possessed by a terror, though no one dares frame it that way.
Bianca's mother, you see, has claustrophobia, a terrible case, and it was agreed
that for her to sleep in their cramped trailer would be painful, insupportable really,
so Bianca's beautiful mother, lusher even than Bianca, and so young seen from here,

younger than my daughter now, would kiss her impassive, pipe-smoking husband
and leave in the car that came every night to take her to the circus-owner's yacht,
and we remnants, we relics, would gloomily sit; Bianca because soon she'd have to go
back to her job as a nightclub dancer, and the husband, for obvious reasons, and me,

part of the act now, with my rituals of desire and my dread of the lions I'll pass again
as I wend the torturous route to my room to wait for Bianca's next visit tomorrow,
with her breasts, and that other thing I could hardly bring myself in those days
to call by its name, so fearsome it was, as it was for the tragic and timid Schulz,

who even in his erotic etchings of perfectly formed nudes with Schulz-like men
abjectly grovelling, crushed, dejected, under their elegant feet, depicts no vaginas,
or none not submerged in inkiest shadow, save one, and that sketchy, inconsequential,
which surely proves that Schulz knew the firmament of vagina is fathomless,

without measurable dimensions, altering such shape it does have with impatience,
but for which Schulz's Bianca, who 'controlled her glamour with pity',
and whose wisdom was 'full of sadness', must by now offer demure consolation,
while mine, my Bianca, struts with top-hat and whip across the arena to take her bow.

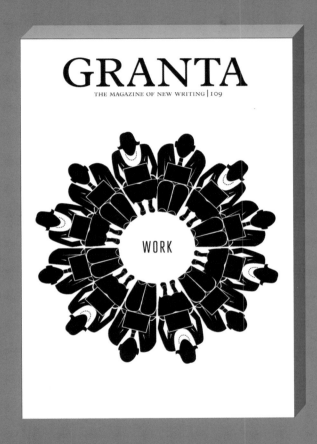

EMPTY PORN SETS

Jo Broughton

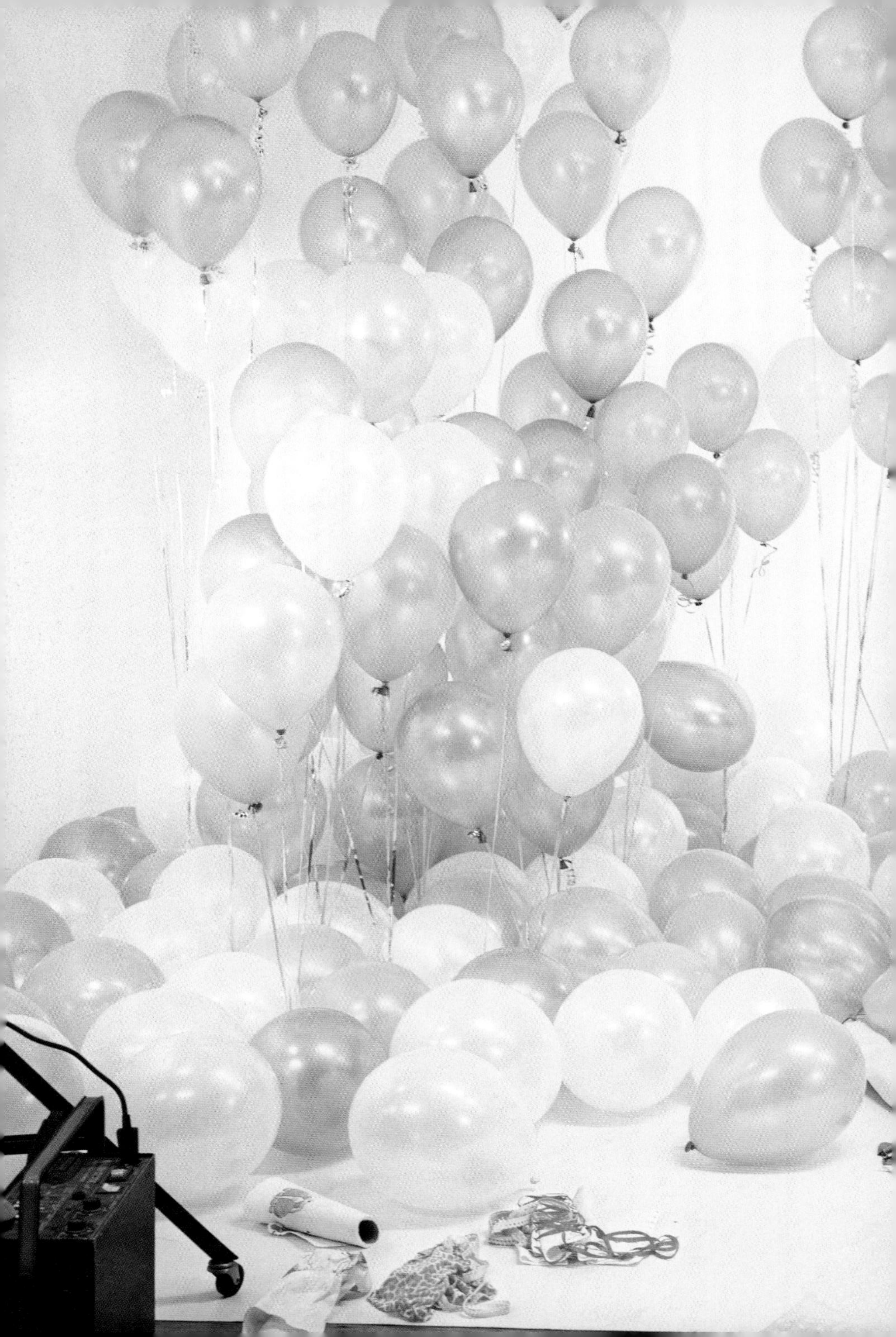

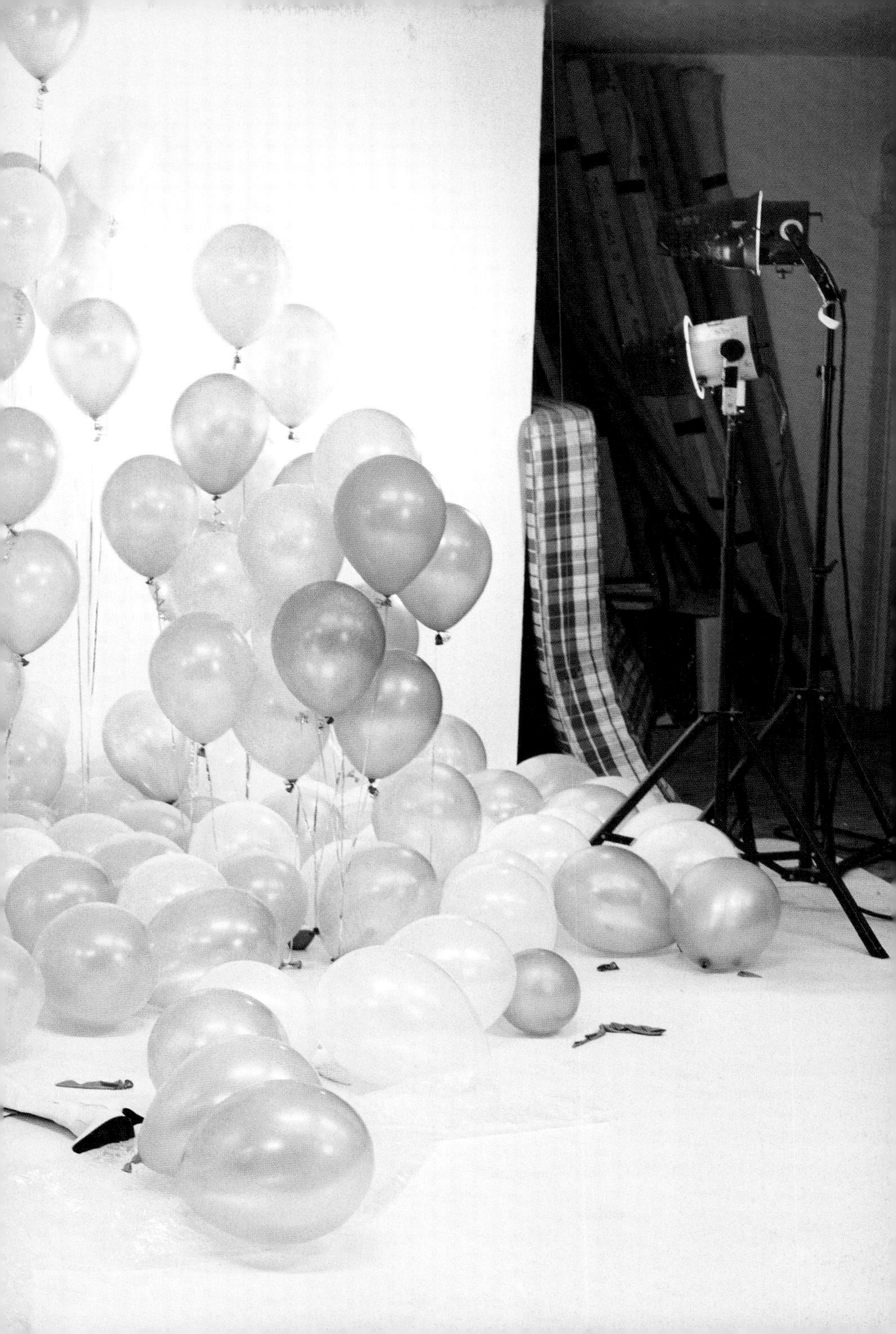

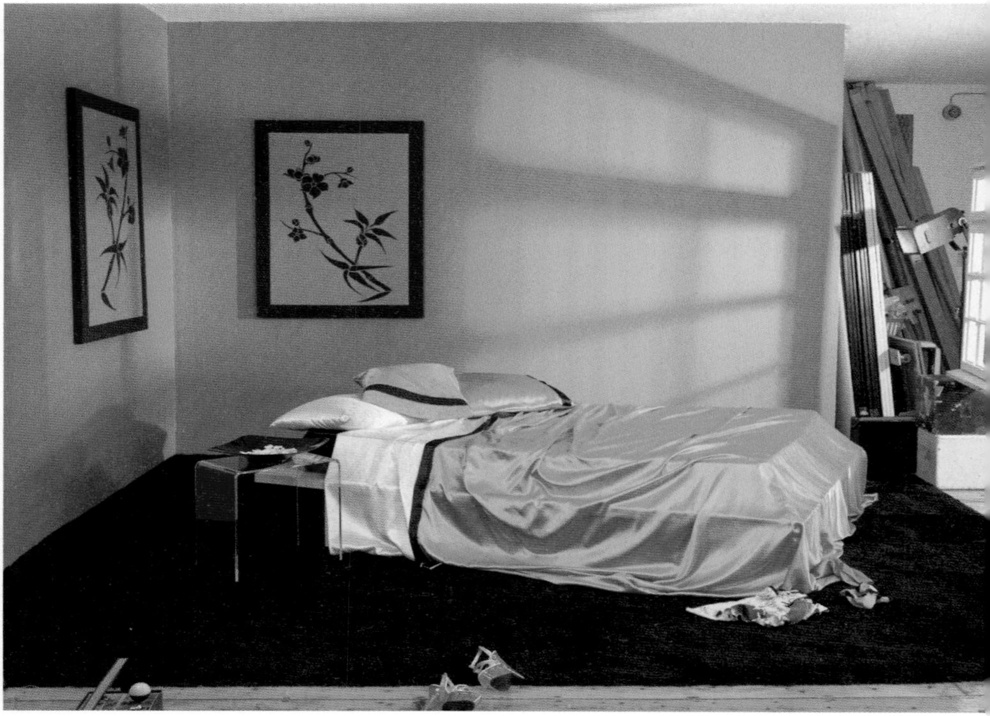

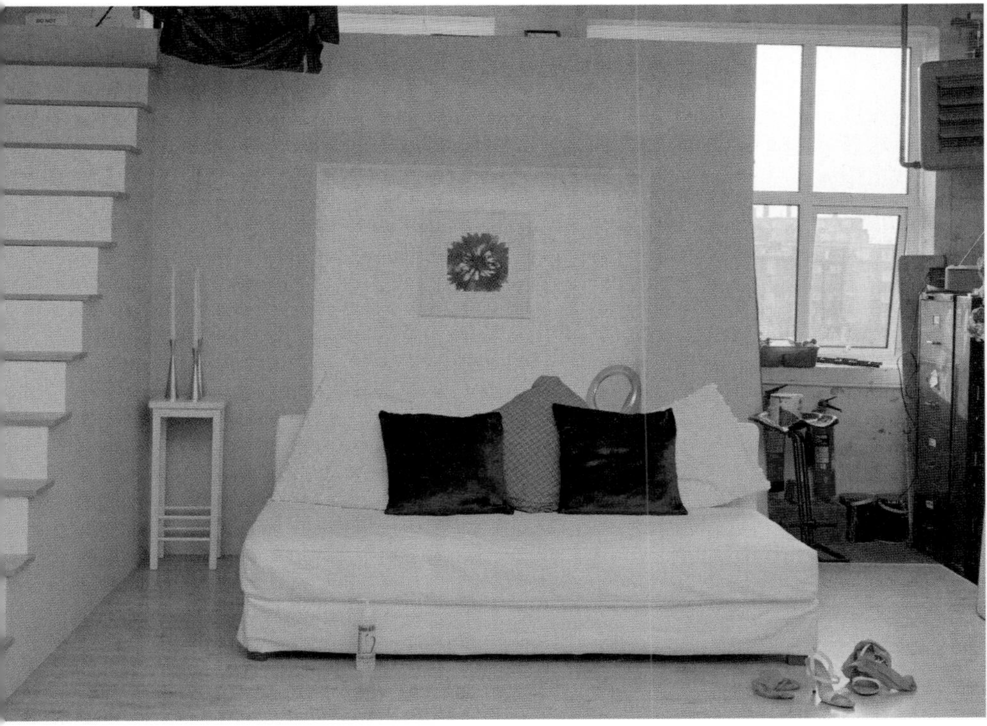

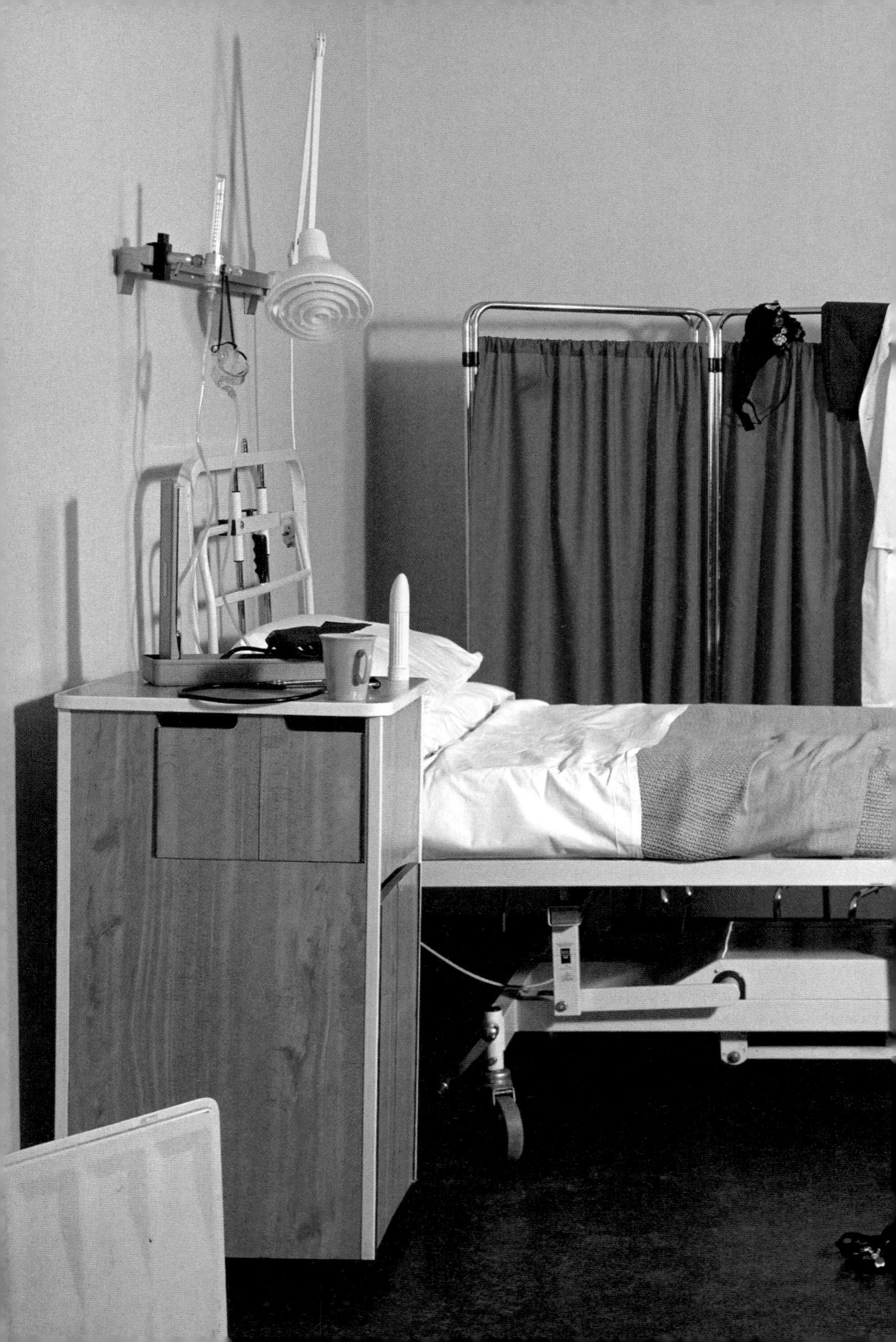

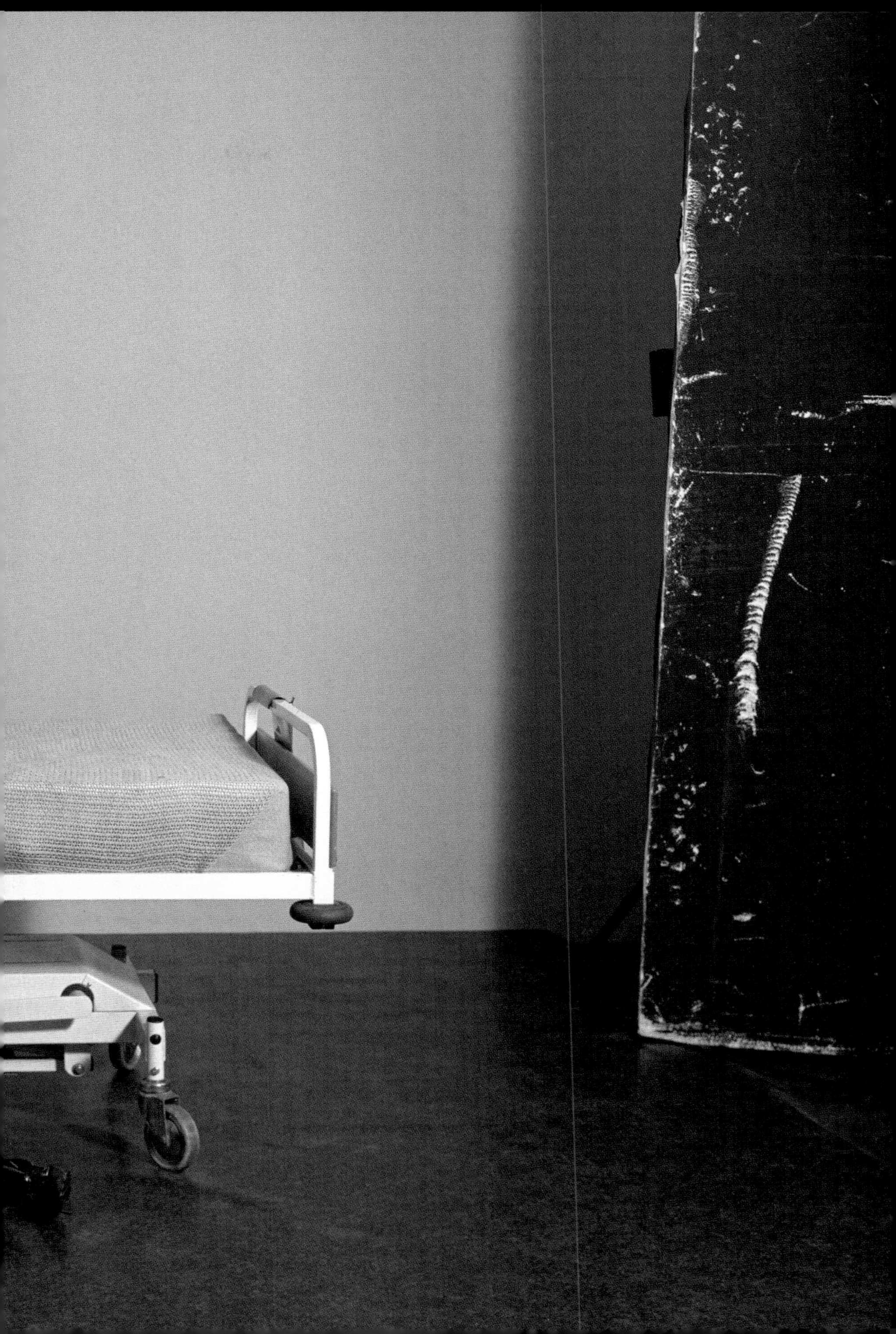

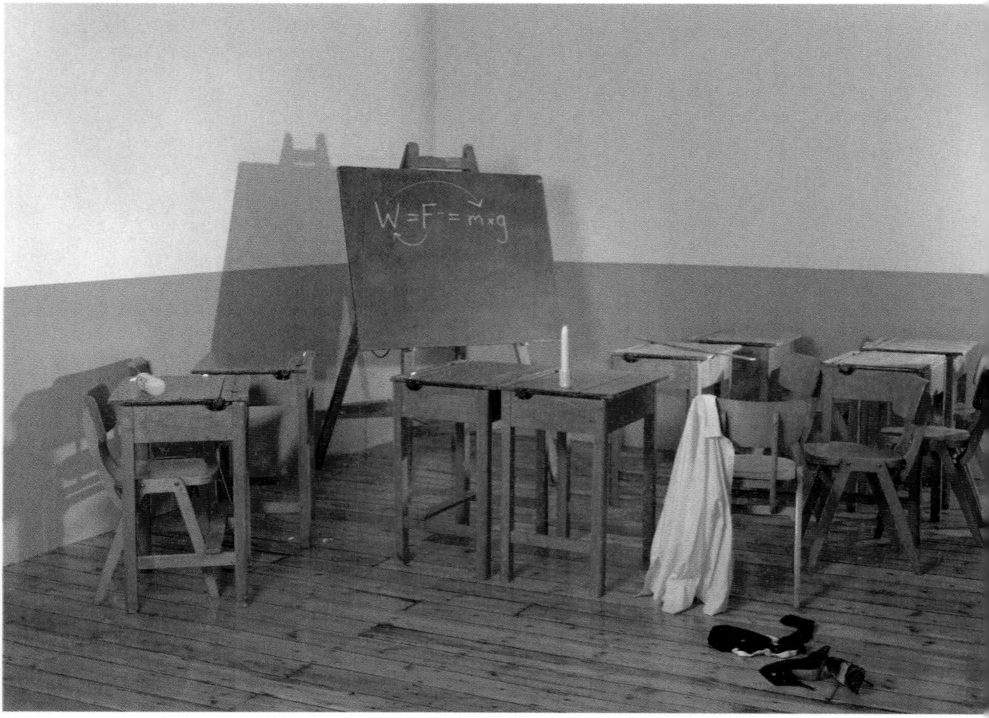
W = F = m×g

THE GOLD CURE

Jennifer Egan

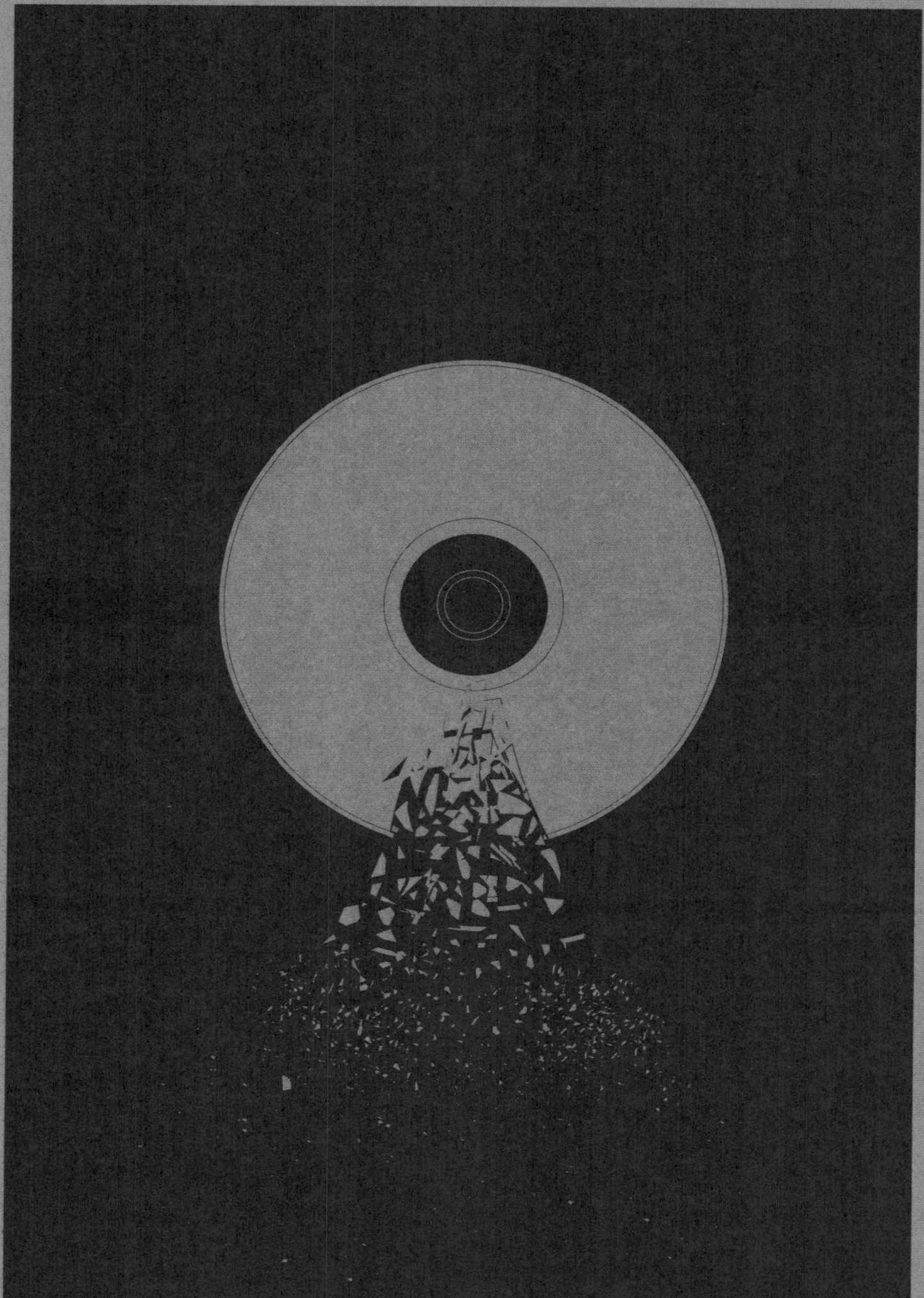

The shame memories began early that day for Bennie, during the morning meeting, while he listened to one of his senior executives make a case for pulling the plug on Stop/Go, a sister band Bennie had signed to a three-record deal a couple of years back. Stop/Go had seemed like an excellent bet; the sisters were young and adorable, their sound was gritty and simple and catchy ('Cyndi Lauper meets Chrissie Hynde' had been Bennie's line early on), with a big gulping bass and some fun percussion – he recalled a cowbell. Plus they'd written decent songs; hell, they'd sold 12,000 CDs off the stage before Bennie ever heard them play. A little time to develop potential singles, some clever marketing and a decent video could put them over the top.

But the sisters were now pushing thirty, his executive producer, Collette, informed Bennie, and were no longer credible as recent high-school grads, especially since one of them had a nine-year-old daughter. Their band members were in law school. They'd fired two producers and a third had quit. Still no album.

'Who's managing them?' Bennie asked.

'Their father. I've got their new rough mix,' Collette said. 'The vocals are buried under seven layers of guitar.'

It was then that the memory overcame Bennie (had the word 'sisters' brought it on?): himself, squatting behind a nunnery in Westchester at sunrise after a night of partying – twenty years ago was it? More? Hearing waves of pure, ringing, spooky-sweet sound waft into the paling sky: cloistered nuns who saw no one but each other, who'd taken vows of silence, singing the Mass. Wet grass under his knees, its iridescence throbbing against his exhausted eyeballs. Even now, Bennie could hear the unearthly sweetness of those nuns' voices echoing deep in his ears.

He'd set up a meeting with their Mother Superior – the only nun you could talk to – brought along a couple of girls from the office for camouflage and waited in a kind of anteroom until the Mother Superior appeared behind a square opening in the wall, like a window without glass. She wore all white, a cloth tightly encircling her face. Bennie remembered her laughing a lot, rosy cheeks lifting into swags, maybe from joy at the thought of bringing God into millions of homes, maybe at the novelty of an A & R guy in purple corduroy making his pitch. The deal was done in a matter of minutes.

He'd approached the cut-out square to say goodbye (here Bennie thrashed in his conference-room chair, anticipating the moment it was all leading up to). The Mother Superior leaned forward slightly, tilting her head in a way that must have triggered something in Bennie, because he lurched across the sill and kissed her on the mouth: velvety skin-fuzz, an intimate, baby-powder smell in the half-second before the nun cried out and jerked away. Then pulling back, grinning through his dread, seeing her appalled, injured face.

'Bennie?' Collette was standing in front of a console, holding the Stop/Go CD. Everyone seemed to be waiting. 'You want to hear this?'

But Bennie was caught in a loop from twenty years before: lungeing over the sill toward the Mother Superior like some haywire figure on a clock, again. Again. Again.

'No,' he groaned. He turned his sweating face into the rivery breeze that gusted through the windows of the old Tribeca coffee factory where Sow's Ear Records occupied two floors. He'd never recorded the nuns. By the time he'd returned from the convent, a message had been waiting.

'I don't,' he told Collette. 'I don't want to hear the mix.' He felt shaken, soiled. Bennie dropped artists all the time; sometimes three in a week, but now his own shame tinged the Stop/Go sisters' failure, as if *he* were to blame. And that feeling was followed by a restless, opposing need to recall what had first excited him about the sisters – to feel that excitement again. 'Why don't I visit them?' he said suddenly.

Collette looked startled, then suspicious, and then worried, a succession that would have amused Bennie if he hadn't been so rattled. 'Really?' she asked.

'Sure. I'll do it today, after I see my kid.'

Bennie's assistant, Sasha, brought him coffee: cream and two sugars. He shimmied a tiny red enamelled box from his pocket, popped the tricky latch, pinched a few gold flakes between his trembling fingers and released them into his cup. He'd begun this regimen two months ago, after reading in a book on Aztec medicine that gold and coffee together were believed to ensure sexual potency. Bennie's goal was more basic than potency: sex *drive*, his own having mysteriously expired. He wasn't sure quite when or quite why this had happened: the divorce from Stephanie? The battle over Christopher? Having recently turned forty-four? Stage one of a devouring illness?

The gold landed on the coffee's milky surface and spun wildly. Bennie was mesmerized by this spinning, which he took as evidence of the explosive gold/coffee chemistry. A frenzy of activity that had mostly led him in circles: wasn't that a fairly accurate description of lust? At times Bennie didn't even mind its disappearance; it was sort of a relief not to be constantly wanting to fuck someone. The world was unquestionably a more peaceful place without the half hard-on that had been his constant companion since the age of thirteen, but did Bennie want to live in such a world? He sipped his gold-inflected coffee and glanced at Sasha's breasts, which had become the litmus test he used to gauge his improvement. He'd lusted after her for most of the years she'd worked for him, first as an intern, then a receptionist, finally his assistant (where she'd remained, oddly reluctant to become an executive in her own right) – and she'd somehow managed to elude that lust without ever saying no, or hurting Bennie's feelings, or pissing him off. And now: Sasha's breasts in a thin yellow sweater, and Bennie felt nothing. Not a shiver of harmless excitement. Could he even get it up if he wanted to?

Driving to pick up his son, Bennie alternated between the Sleepers and the Dead Kennedys, San Francisco bands he'd grown up with. He listened for the muddiness, the sense of actual musicians playing actual instruments in an actual room. Nowadays that quality (if it existed at all) was usually an effect of analogue signalling rather than real tape – everything was an effect in the bloodless constructions Bennie and his peers were churning out. He worked tirelessly, feverishly, to get things right, stay on top, make songs that people would love and buy and download as ringtones (and steal, of course) – above all, to satisfy the multinational crude-oil extractors he'd sold his label to five years ago. But Bennie knew that what he was bringing into the world was shit. Too clear, too clean. The problem was precision, perfection; the problem was *digitization*, which sucked the life out of everything that got smeared through its microscopic mesh. Film, photography, music: dead. *An aesthetic holocaust!* Bennie knew better than to say these things aloud.

But the deep thrill of these old songs lay, for Bennie, in the rapturous surges of sixteen-year-old-ness they induced; Bennie and his high school gang – Scotty and Alice, Jocelyn and Rhea – all of whom he was decades out of touch with (except for a disturbing encounter with Scotty in his office, years ago), yet still half believed he'd find waiting in line outside the Mabuhay Gardens (long-defunct), in San Francisco, green-haired and safety-pinned, if he happened to show up there one Saturday night.

And then, as Jello Biafra was thrashing his way through 'Too Drunk to Fuck', Bennie's mind drifted to an awards ceremony a few years ago where he'd tried to introduce a jazz pianist as 'incomparable' and ended up calling her 'incompetent' before an audience of 2,500. He should never have tried for 'incomparable' – wasn't his word, too fancy; it stuck in his mouth every time he'd practised his speech for Stephanie. But it suited the pianist, who had miles of shiny gold hair, and had also (she'd let slip) graduated from Harvard. Bennie had cherished a wild dream of getting her into bed, feeling that hair sliding over his shoulders and chest.

He idled now in front of Christopher's school, waiting for the memory spasm to pass. Driving in, he'd glimpsed his son crossing the athletic field with his friends. Chris had been skipping a little –

actually skipping – tossing a ball in the air, but by the time he slumped into Bennie's yellow Porsche, any inkling of lightness was gone. Why? Did Chris somehow know about the botched awards ceremony? Bennie told himself this was nuts, yet was seized by an urge to confess the malapropism to his fourth-grader. The Will to Divulge, Dr Beet called this impulse, and had exhorted Bennie to write down the things he wanted to confide, rather than burden his son with them. Bennie did this now, scribbling 'incompetent' on the back of a parking ticket he'd received the day before. Then, recalling the earlier humiliation, he added to the list 'kissing Mother Superior'.

'So, boss,' he said. 'Whatcha feel like doing?'

'Don't know.'

'Any paticular wishes?'

'Not really.'

Bennie looked helplessly out the window. A couple of months ago, Chris had asked if they could skip their weekly appointment with Dr Beet and spend the afternoon 'doing whatever' instead. They hadn't gone back, a decision that Bennie now regretted; 'doing whatever' had led to desultory afternoons, often cut short by Chris's announcement that he had homework.

'How about some coffee?' Bennie suggested.

A spark of smile. 'Can I get a Frappuccino?'

'Don't tell your mother.'

Stephanie didn't approve of Chris drinking coffee – reasonable, given that the kid was nine – but Bennie couldn't resist the exquisite connection that came of defying his ex-wife in unison. Betrayal Bonding, Dr Beet called this and, like the Will to Divulge, it was on the list of no-nos.

They got their coffees and returned to the Porsche to drink them. Chris sucked greedily at his Frappuccino. Bennie took out his red enamelled box, pinched a few gold flakes, and slipped them under the plastic lid of his cup.

'What's that?' Chris asked.

Bennie started. The gold was becoming so routine that he'd

stopped being clandestine about it. 'Medicine,' he said, after a moment.

'For what?'

'Some symptoms I've been having.' *Or not having*, he added mentally.

'What symptoms?'

Was this the Frappuccino kicking in? Chris had shifted out of his slump and now sat upright, regarding Bennie with his wide, dark, frankly beautiful eyes. 'Headaches,' Bennie said.

'Can I see it?' Chris asked. 'The medicine? In that red thing?'

Bennie handed over the lacquered box. Within a couple of seconds, the kid had figured out the tricky latch and popped it open. 'Whoa, Dad,' he said. 'What is this stuff?'

'I told you.'

'It looks like gold. Flakes of gold.'

'It has a flaky consistency.'

'Can I taste one?'

'Son. You don't –'

'Just one?'

Bennie sighed. 'One.'

The boy carefully removed a gold flake and placed it on his tongue. 'What does it taste like?' Bennie couldn't help asking. He'd only consumed the gold in his coffee, where it had no discernible flavour.

'Like metal,' Chris said. 'It's awesome. Can I have another one?'

Bennie started the car. Was there something obviously sham about the medicine story? Clearly the kid wasn't buying it. 'One more,' he said. 'And that's it.'

His son took a fat pinch of gold flakes and put them on his tongue. Bennie tried not to think of the money. The truth was, he'd spent $8,000 on gold in the past two months. A coke habit would have cost him less.

Chris sucked on the gold and closed his eyes. 'Dad,' he said, 'it's, like, waking me up from the inside.'

'Interesting,' Bennie mused. 'That's exactly what it's supposed to do.'

'Is it working?'

'Sounds like it is.'

'But on you,' Chris said.

Bennie was fairly certain his son had asked him more questions in the past ten minutes than in the year and a half since he and Stephanie had split. Could this be a side effect of the gold: curiosity?

'I've still got the headaches,' he said.

He was driving aimlessly among the Crandale mansions ('doing whatever' involved a lot of aimless driving), every one of which seemed to have four or five blond children in Ralph Lauren playing out front. Seeing these kids, it was clearer than ever to Bennie that he hadn't had a chance of lasting in this place, swarthy and unkempt-looking as he was even when freshly showered and shaved. Stephanie, meanwhile, had ascended to the club's number-one doubles team.

'Chris,' Bennie said, 'there's a musical group I need to visit – a pair of young sisters. Well, youngish sisters. I was planning to go later on, but if you're interested, we could –'

'Sure.'

'Really?'

'Yeah.'

Did 'sure' and 'yeah' mean that Chris was giving in to please Bennie, as Dr Beet had noted he often did? Or had the gold-incited curiosity extended to a new interest in Bennie's work? Chris had grown up around rock groups, but he was part of the post-piracy generation, for whom things like 'copyright' and 'creative ownership' didn't exist. Bennie didn't *blame* Chris, of course; the dismantlers who had murdered the music business were a generation beyond his son, adults now. Still, he'd heeded Dr Beet's advice to stop hectoring (Beet's word) Chris about the industry's decline, and focus instead on enjoying music they both liked – Pearl Jam, for example, which Bennie blasted all the way to Mount Vernon.

The Stop/Go sisters still lived with their parents in a sprawling, run-down house under bushy suburban trees. Bennie had been here two or three years ago when he'd first discovered them, before he'd entrusted the sisters to the first in a series of executives who had failed to accomplish a blessed thing. As he and Chris left the car, the memory of his last visit provoked a convulsion of anger in Bennie that made heat roll up toward his head – why the fuck hadn't anything happened in all this time?

He found Sasha waiting at the door; she'd caught the train at Grand Central after Bennie called and had somehow beaten him here.

'Hiya, Crisco,' Sasha said, mussing his son's hair. She had known Chris all his life; she'd run out to Duane Reade to buy him pacifiers and diapers. Bennie glanced at her breasts; nothing. Or nothing sexual – he did feel a swell of gratitude and appreciation for his assistant, as opposed to the murderous rage he felt toward the rest of his staff.

There was a pause. Yellow light scissored through the leaves. Bennie lifted his gaze from Sasha's breasts to her face. She had high cheekbones and narrow green eyes, wavy hair that ranged from reddish to purplish, depending on the month. Today it was red. She was smiling at Chris, but Bennie detected worry somewhere in the smile. He rarely thought of Sasha as an independent person, and beyond a vague awareness of boyfriends coming and going (vague first out of respect for her privacy, lately out of indifference), he knew few specifics of her life. But seeing her outside this family home, Bennie experienced a flare of curiosity: Sasha had been a student at NYU when he'd first met her at a Conduits gig at the Pyramid Club; that put her in her thirties now. Why hadn't she married? Did she want kids? She seemed suddenly older, or was it just that Bennie seldom looked directly at her face?

'What?' she said, feeling his stare.

'Nothing.'

'You OK?'

'Better than OK,' Bennie said, and gave the door a sharp knock.

The sisters looked fantastic – if not right out of high school then at least right out of college, especially if they'd taken a year or two off or maybe transferred a couple of times. They wore their dark hair pulled back from their faces, and their eyes were glittering, and they had a whole fucking book full of new material – *look at this*! Bennie's fury at his team intensified, but it was pleasurable, motivating fury. The sisters' nervous excitement jittered up the house; they knew his visit was their last, best hope. Chandra was the older one, Louisa the younger. Louisa's daughter, Olivia, had been riding a trike in the driveway on Bennie's last visit, but now she wore skintight jeans and a jewelled tiara that seemed to be a fashion choice, not a costume. Bennie felt Chris snap to attention when Olivia entered the room.

They went single file down a narrow flight of stairs to the sisters' basement recording studio. Their father had built it for them years ago. It was tiny, with orange shag covering the floor, ceiling and walls. Bennie took the only seat, noting with approval a cowbell by the keyboard.

'Coffee?' Sasha asked him. Chandra led her upstairs to make it. Louisa sat at the keyboard teasing out melodies. Olivia took up a set of bongo drums and began loosely accompanying her mother. She handed Chris a tambourine, and to Bennie's surprise, his son settled in beating the thing in perfect time. Nice, he thought. Very nice. The day had swerved unexpectedly into good. The almost-teenage daughter wasn't a problem, he decided; she could join the group as a younger sister or a cousin, strengthen the tween angle. Maybe Chris could be part of it, too, although he and Olivia would have to switch instruments. A boy on a tambourine ...

Sasha brought his coffee, and Bennie took out his red lacquered box and dropped in a pinch of flakes. As he sipped, a sensation of pleasure filled his whole torso the way a snowfall fills up a sky. Jesus, he felt good. He'd been delegating too much. Hearing the music get *made*, that was the thing: people and instruments and beaten-looking equipment aligning abruptly into a single structure of sound, flexible and alive. The sisters were at the keyboard arranging their music, and Bennie experienced a bump of anticipation; something was going to happen, here. He knew it. Felt it pricking his arms and chest.

'You've got Pro-Tools on there, right?' he asked, indicating the laptop on a table amid the instruments. 'Is everything miked? Can we lay down some tracks right now?'

The sisters nodded and checked the laptop; they were ready to record. 'Vocals, too?' Chandra asked.

'Absolutely,' Bennie said. 'Let's do it all at once. Let's blow the roof off your fucking house.'

Sasha was standing to Bennie's right. So many bodies had heated up the little room, lifting off her skin a perfume she'd been wearing for years – or was it a lotion? – that smelled like apricots; not just the sweet part but that slight bitterness around the pit. And as Bennie breathed in Sasha's lotion smell, his prick roused itself suddenly like an old hound getting a swift kick. He almost jumped out of his seat in startled amazement, but he kept his cool. Don't push things, just let it happen. Don't scare it away.

Then the sisters began to sing. Oh, the raw, almost threadbare sound of their voices mixed with the throb and smash of instruments – these sensations met with a faculty deeper in Bennie than judgement or even pleasure; they communed directly with his body, whose shivering, bursting reply made him dizzy. And here was his first erection in months – prompted by Sasha, who had been too near Bennie all these years for him really to see her, like in those nineteenth-century novels he'd read in secret because only girls were supposed to like them. Bennie seized the cowbell and stick and began whacking at it with zealous blows. He felt the music in his mouth, his ears, his ribs – or was that his own pulse? He was on fire!

And from this zenith of lusty, devouring joy, he recalled opening an e-mail he'd been inadvertently copied in on between two colleagues and finding himself referred to as a 'hairball'. God, what a feeling of liquid shame had pooled in Bennie when he'd read that word. He hadn't been sure what it meant: that he was hairy (true)? Unclean (false!)? Or was it literal, as in: he clogged people's throats and made them gag, the way Stephanie's cat, Sylph, occasionally vomited hair onto the carpet? He'd gone for a haircut that very day and seriously considered having his back and upper arms waxed, until Stephanie talked him out of it, running her cool hands over his shoulders that night in bed, telling him she loved him hairy – that the last thing the world needed was another waxed guy.

Music. Bennie was listening to music. The sisters were screaming, the tiny room imploding from their sound, and Bennie tried to find again the deep contentment he'd felt just a minute ago. But 'hairball' had unsettled him. The room felt uncomfortably small. Bennie set down his cowbell and slipped the parking ticket from his pocket. He scribbled 'hairball' in hopes of exorcizing the memory. He inhaled slowly and rested his eyes on Chris, who was flailing the tambourine trying to match the sisters' erratic tempo, and right away it happened again. Taking his son for a haircut a couple of years ago, having his long-time barber, Stu, put down his scissors and pull Bennie aside. 'There's a problem with your son's hair,' he'd said.

'A problem?'

Stu walked Bennie over to Chris in the chair and parted his hair to reveal some tan little creatures the size of poppy seeds moving around on his scalp. Bennie felt himself grow faint. 'Lice,' the barber whispered. 'They get it at school.'

'But he goes to private school!' Bennie had blurted. 'In Crandale, New York!'

Chris's eyes had gone wide with fear: 'What is it, Daddy?' Other people were staring, and Bennie had felt responsible, with his own riotous head of hair, to the point where he sprayed OFF! in his armpits every morning to this day, kept an extra can at the office – crazy! He knew it. Getting their coats while everyone watched, Bennie with a burning face; God, it hurt him to think of this now – hurt him physically, as if the memory were raking over him and leaving gashes. He hid his face in his hands. He wanted to cover his ears, block out the cacophony of Stop/Go, but he concentrated on Sasha, just to his right, her sweet/bitter smell, and found himself remembering a girl he'd chased at a party when he'd first come to New York and was selling vinyl on the Lower East Side a hundred years ago, some delicious blonde – Abby was it? In the course of keeping tabs on Abby, Bennie had done several lines of coke and been stricken with a severe and instantaneous need to empty his bowels. He'd been relieving himself on the can in what must have been (although Bennie's brain ached to recall this) a miasma of annihilating stink, when the unlockable bathroom door had jumped open and there was Abby, staring down at him. There'd been a horrible, bottomless instant when their eyes met; then she'd shut the door.

Bennie had left the party with someone else – there was always someone else – and their night of fun, which he felt comfortable presuming, had erased the confrontation with Abby. But now it was back – oh, it was back, bringing waves of shame so immense they seemed to engulf whole parts of Bennie's life and haul them away: achievements, successes, moments of pride, all of it razed to the point where there was nothing – *he* was nothing – but a guy on a john looking up at the nauseated face of a woman he'd wanted to impress.

Bennie leapt from his stool, squashing the cowbell under one foot. Sweat stung his eyes. His hair engaged palpably with the ceiling shag.

'You OK?' Sasha asked, alarmed.

'I'm sorry,' Bennie panted, mopping his brow. 'I'm sorry. I'm sorry. I'm sorry.'

Back upstairs, he stood outside the front door, pulling fresh air into his lungs. The Stop/Go sisters and daughter clustered around him, apologizing for the airlessness of the recording studio, their father's ongoing failure to vent it properly, reminding each other in spirited tones of the many times they themselves had grown faint, trying to work there.

'We can hum the tunes,' they said, and they did, in harmony, Olivia too, all of them standing not far from Bennie's face, desperation quivering their smiles. A grey cat made a figure eight around Bennie's shins, nudging him rapturously with its bony head. It was a relief to get back in the car.

He was driving Sasha to the city, but he had to get Chris home first. His son hunched in the back seat, facing the open window. It seemed to Bennie that his lark of an idea for the afternoon had gone awry. He fended off the impulse to look at Sasha's breasts, waiting to calm down, regain his equilibrium before putting himself to the test. Finally, at a red light, he glanced slowly, casually in her direction, not even focusing at first, then peering intently. Nothing. He was clobbered by loss so severe that it took physical effort not to howl. He'd had it, *he'd had it*! But where had it gone?

'Dad. Green light,' Chris said.

Driving again, Bennie forced himself to ask his son, 'So, boss. What did you think?'

The kid didn't answer. Maybe he was pretending not to hear, or maybe the wind was too loud in his face. Bennie glanced at Sasha. 'What about you?'

'Oh,' she said, 'they're awful.'

Bennie blinked, stung. He felt a swell of anger at Sasha that passed a few seconds later, leaving odd relief. Of course. They were awful. That was the problem.

'Unlistenable,' Sasha went on. 'No wonder you were having a heart attack.'

'I don't get it,' Bennie said.

'What?'

'Two years ago they sounded … different.'

Sasha gave him a quizzical look. 'It wasn't two years,' she said. 'It was five.'

'Why so sure?'

'Because last time, I came to their house after a meeting at Windows on the World.'

It took Bennie a minute to comprehend this. 'Oh,' he finally said. 'How close to ...?'

'Four days.'

'Wow. I never knew that.' He waited out a respectful pause, then continued. 'Still, two years, five years ...'

Sasha turned and stared at him. She looked angry. 'Who am I talking to?' she asked. 'You're Bennie Salazar! This is the music business. "Five years is five *hundred* years" – your words.'

Bennie didn't answer. They were approaching his former house, as he thought of it. He couldn't say 'old house', but he also couldn't say 'house' anymore, although he'd certainly paid for it. His former house was withdrawn from the street on a grassy slope; a gleaming white colonial that had filled him with awe every time he'd taken a key from his pocket to open the front door. Bennie stopped at the kerb and killed the engine. He couldn't bring himself to drive up the driveway.

Chris was leaning forward from the back seat, his head between Bennie and Sasha. Bennie wasn't sure how long he'd been there. 'I think you need some of your medicine, Dad,' he said.

'Good idea,' Bennie said. He began tapping his pockets, but the little red box was nowhere to be found.

'Here, I've got it,' Sasha said. 'You dropped it coming out of the recording room.'

She was doing that more and more, finding things he'd misplaced – sometimes before Bennie even knew they were missing. It added to the almost trance-like dependence he felt on her. 'Thanks, Sash,' he said.

He opened the box. God the flakes were shiny. Gold didn't tarnish, that was the thing. The flakes would look the same in five years as they did right now.

'Should I put some on my tongue, like you did?' he asked his son.

'Yeah. But I get some too.'

'Sasha, you want to try a little medicine?' Bennie asked.

'Um, OK,' she said. 'What's it supposed to do?'

'Solve your problems,' Bennie said. 'I mean, headaches. Not that you have any.'

'Never,' Sasha said, with that same wary smile.

They each took a pinch of gold flakes and placed it on their tongues. Bennie tried not to calculate the dollar value of what was inside their mouths. He concentrated on the taste: was it metallic, or was that just his expectation? Coffee, or was that what was left in his mouth? He tongued the gold in a tight knot and sucked the juice from within it; sour, he thought. Bitter. Sweet? Each one seemed true for a second, but in the end Bennie had an impression of something mineral, like stone. Even earth. And then the lump melted away.

'I should go, Dad,' Chris said. Bennie let him out of the car and hugged him hard. As always, Chris went still in his embrace, but whether he was savouring it or enduring it Bennie could never tell.

He drew back and looked at his son. The baby he and Stephanie had nuzzled and kissed – now this painful, mysterious presence. Bennie had an urge to say, 'Don't tell your mother about the medicine,' craving an instant of connection with Chris before he went inside. But he hesitated, employing a mental calculation Dr Beet had taught him: did he really think the kid would tell Stephanie about the gold? No. And that was his alert: Betrayal Bonding. Bennie said nothing.

He got back in the car, but didn't turn the key. He was watching Chris scale the undulating lawn toward his former house. The grass was fluorescently bright. His son seemed to buckle under his enormous backpack. What the hell was in it? Bennie had seen professional photographers carry less. As Chris neared the house he blurred a little, or maybe it was Bennie's eyes watering. He found it excruciating, watching his son's long journey to the front door. He worried Sasha would speak – say something like, 'He's a great kid,' or, 'That was fun,' something that would require Bennie to turn and look at her. But Sasha knew better; she knew everything. She sat with Bennie in silence, watching Chris climb the fat, bright grass to the front door, then open it without turning and go inside.

They didn't speak again until they'd passed from the Henry Hudson Parkway on to the West Side Highway, heading into lower Manhattan. Bennie played some early Who, the Stooges, bands he'd listened to before he was old enough to go to a concert. Then he got into the Mutants, Eye Protection – seventies Bay Area groups he and his gang had slam-danced to at the Mabuhay Gardens when they weren't practising with their own unlistenable band, the Flaming Dildos. He sensed Sasha paying attention, and toyed with the idea that he was confessing to her his disillusionment – his *hatred* for the industry he'd given his life to. He began weighing each musical choice, drawing out his argument through the songs themselves – Patti Smith's ragged poetry (but why did she quit?), the jock hardcore of Black Flag and the Circle Jerks giving way to Alternative, that great compromise, down, down, down to the singles he'd just today been petitioning radio stations to add, husks of music, lifeless and cold as the squares of office neon cutting the blue twilight.

'It's incredible,' Sasha said, 'how there's just nothing there.'

Astounded, Bennie turned to her. Was it possible that she'd followed his musical rant to its grim conclusion? Sasha was looking downtown, and he followed her eyes to the empty space where the Twin Towers had been. 'There should be *something*, you know?' she said, not looking at Bennie. 'Like an echo. Or an outline.'

Bennie sighed. 'They'll put something up,' he said. 'When they're finally done squabbling.'

'I know.' But she kept looking south, as if it were a problem her mind couldn't solve. Bennie was relieved she hadn't understood. He remembered his mentor, Lou Kline, telling him once in the nineties that rock and roll had peaked at Monterey Pop. They'd been in Lou's house in LA with its waterfalls, the pretty girls Lou always had, his car collection out front, and Bennie had looked into his idol's famous face and thought, 'You're finished.' Nostalgia was the end – everyone knew that. Lou had died three months ago, after years of being paralysed from a stroke.

At a stop light, Bennie remembered his list. He took out the parking ticket and finished it off.

'What do you keep scribbling on that ticket?' Sasha asked. Bennie handed it to her, his reluctance to have the list seen by human eyes overwhelming him a half-second late. To his horror, she began reading it aloud:

Kissing Mother Superior
Incompetent
Hairball

Poppy seeds
On the can

Bennie listened in agony, as if the words themselves might provoke a catastrophe. But they were neutralized the instant Sasha spoke them in her scratchy voice.

'Not bad,' she said. 'They're titles, right?'

'Sure,' Bennie said. 'Can you read them one more time?' She did, and now they sounded like titles to him, too. He felt peaceful, cleansed.

'"Kissing Mother Superior" is my favourite,' Sasha said. 'We've gotta find a way to use that one.'

They'd pulled up outside her building, on Forsyth. The street felt desolate and underlit. Bennie wished she could live in a better place. Sasha gathered up her ubiquitous black bag, a shapeless wishing well from which she'd managed to wrest whatever file or number or slip of paper he'd needed for the past twelve years. Bennie seized her thin pale hand. 'Listen,' he said. 'Listen, Sasha.'

She looked up. Bennie felt no lust at all – he wasn't even hard. What he felt for Sasha was love, a safety and closeness like what he'd had with Stephanie before he'd let her down so many times that she couldn't stop being mad. 'I'm crazy for you, Sasha,' he said. 'Crazy.'

'Come on, Bennie,' Sasha chided lightly. 'None of that.'

He held her hand between both of his. Sasha's fingers were trembly and cold. Her other hand was on the door.

'Wait,' Bennie said. 'Please.'

She turned to him, serious. 'There's no way, Bennie,' she said. 'We need each other.'

They looked at one another in the failing light. The delicate bones of Sasha's face were lightly freckled – it was a girl's face, but she'd stopped being a girl when he wasn't looking.

Sasha leaned over and kissed Bennie's cheek: a chaste kiss, a kiss between brother and sister, mother and son, but Bennie felt the softness of her skin, the warm movement of her breath. Then she was out of the car. She waved to him through the window and said something he didn't catch. Bennie lunged across the empty seat, his face near the glass, staring fixedly as she said it again. Still, he missed it. As he struggled to open the door, Sasha said it once more, mouthing the words extra slowly:

'See. You. Tomorrow.' ■

FOUR ANIMALS CONTEMPLATING SEX

Drawings by Dave Eggers

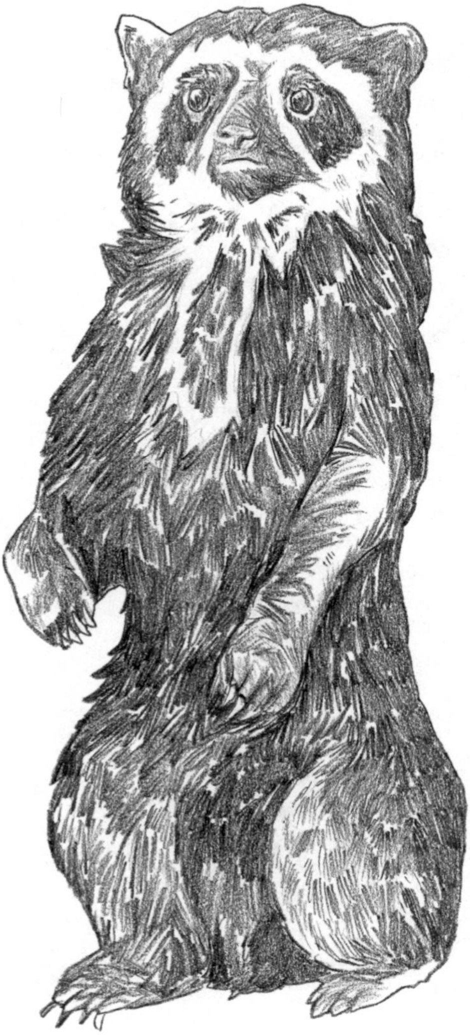

Bespectacled Bear
12 January 2010, 4.51 p.m.

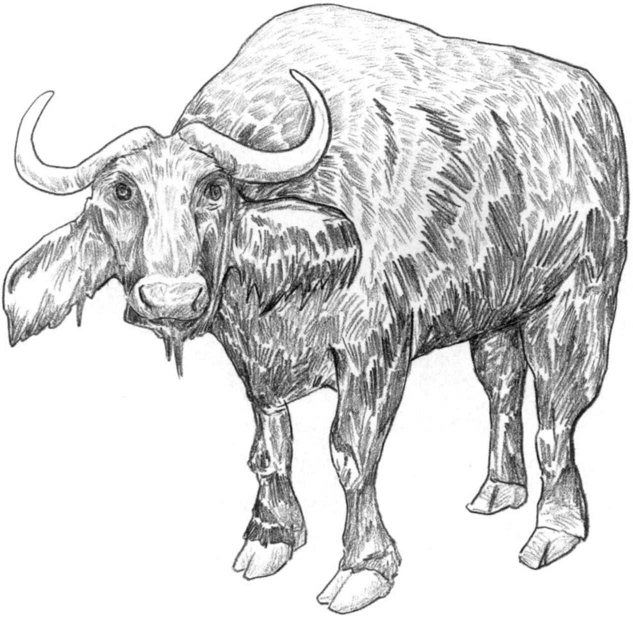

African Buffalo
6 January 2010, 7.10 a.m.

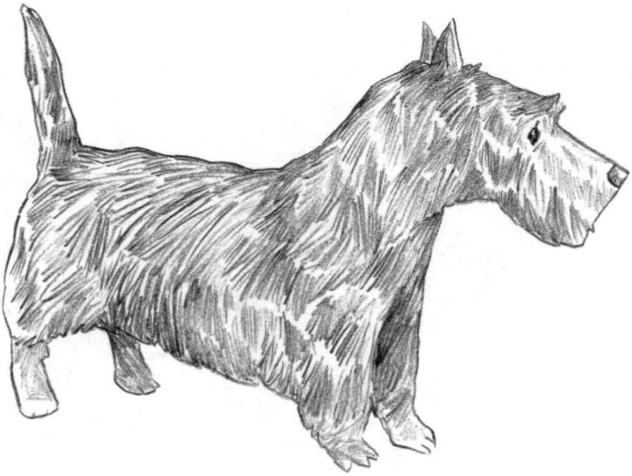

Scottish Terrier
7 January 2010, 1.12 p.m.

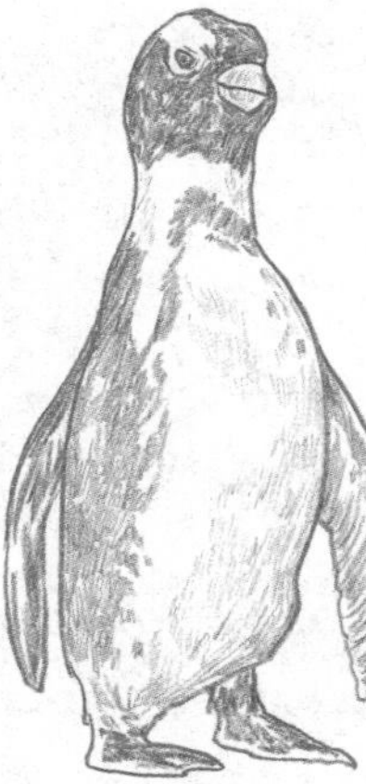

African Penguin
22 January 2010, 5.22 p.m.

SILENCE

Michael Symmons Roberts

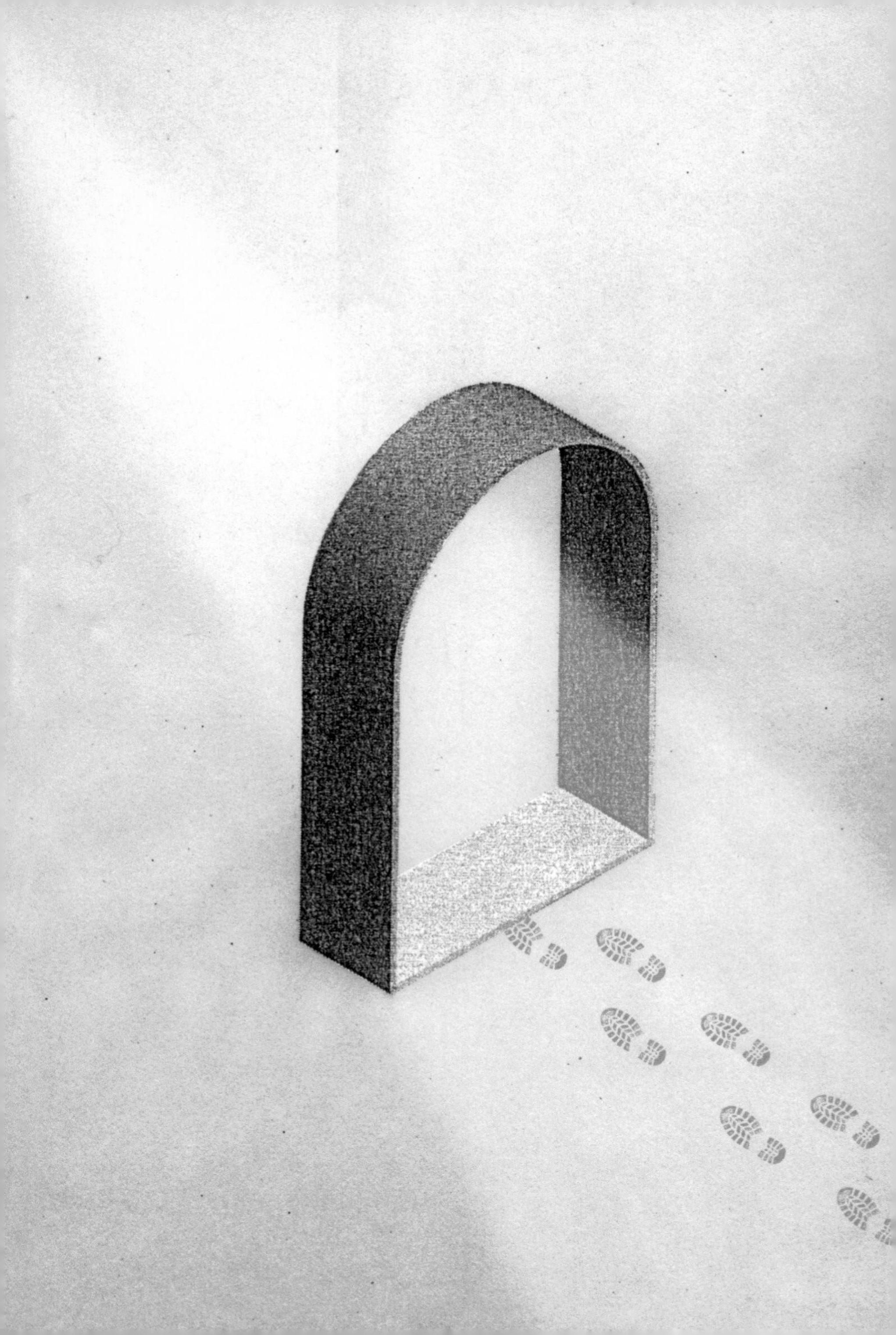

I

A white-robed monk leads me into a modern wing of the monastery. 'There's a board here, which will tell us where you're staying,' he says. We enter a dark hallway. On the board is a column with gold letters listing the rooms. All are named after saints. To the right of each saint's name is a brass slot with a card recording the name of that room's guest. There must be twenty rooms, but there are only two cards in the slots, both handwritten in elegant script. My name is not one of them. 'You don't exist,' says the monk.

A bell rings. I follow him into the abbey where I'm handed a sheet so I can follow the Latin plainsong. The sheet says this service is called 'None'. It is the coldest winter in four decades and I am sitting in the oldest working monastery in Britain, deep in the Scottish Highlands, listening to the oldest music I'm ever likely to hear. It is early afternoon, but 'None' means the ninth hour since the start of the Benedictine day. I do a quick count back, to work out when I'll be getting up tomorrow. I count again, but it's still true.

From the moment my car door slammed across the valley, I was aware of silence here as tangible. Nothing moves in the Glen of the Black Burn. I walk down windowless corridors. Not a trace of anyone. The nave itself, candlelit and cavernous, is a trap to lure the quiet from the hills and hold it. Silence has become incarnate. By the time my name card is written, the word 'None' has got a hold of me. None as in nothing. No one. I've only been here half an hour, but with the absence of people, the bare walls of the monastery and the mile upon mile of frozen white around me, I can feel myself slipping through my fingers.

II

In the early 1950s, W. H. Auden wrote a sequence of poems called *Horae Canonicae*, exploring his own Christian beliefs and following the structure of the monastic day. In his poem about None, there is a chilling section in which he takes you 'To dark chateaux where wind sobs / In the pine-trees and telephones ring, / Inviting trouble, to a room, / Lit by one weak bulb, where our Double sits / Writing and does not look up.'

I like the notion of a study-bedroom, a place where life and work are inseparable, where poems and beliefs can be wrestled with and worked through. I have a postcard at home of St Jerome in his study, resting his head on a hand as he pores over a manuscript. My study here at Pluscarden is simpler than Jerome's. He has a sleeping lion, and a quail pecking at his slippers. And there is a large statue of the crucified Christ looking down on him, to keep him focused on the urgency of his task. Art historians have noted that Jerome's crucifix does not seem to be attached to the desk, and may be a vision. My study here has a crucifix above the bed, but it's not a vision. I've touched it. I also have a sink and a desk. Each time I come back from one of the services, I half expect to find my double sitting at the desk, more real than I am, writing, oblivious to my arrival. I imagine him wearing the white Benedictine habit of the Pluscarden monks.

This is my monastic cell. I walk to the window, and outside, pheasants – vivid and exotic as peacocks against the snow – stalk the grounds in search of scraps. Beyond them, the woods are hunched in afternoon darkness, deep and still. It's snowing again. When I came here, I thought the big issue would be the presence or absence of God, not the presence or absence of me. I think of Auden's poem, and the shattering loneliness of that doppelgänger image. I wonder how long I would have to live a monk's life (chaste, untouched, locked into an endlessly repeated series of rituals) before my mind conjured visions? Auden was about my age – in his mid-forties – when he wrote *Horae Canonicae*. There are twin traditions to the doppelgänger myth.

One suggests that he who meets his double soon meets his death. The other says a meeting with your double is a direct meeting with God. My double has yet to show.

III

As compline comes to an end each night, the monks kneel in front of a statue of Mary, to whom the abbey is dedicated. They look intense, moved, passionately involved in what they are doing. I am moved to watch them, to be transported by the music and the place, but it feels almost indecent to be watching. One by one – as their devotions are finished – they walk out, heads bowed. This is the last office of the monastic day. It is quiet and dark, save for the few tall candles on the altar. The evening plainsong is achingly beautiful, as the community gives thanks for another day and prays for God's blessing and protection through the night. In a service like this one, it is possible to imagine a kind of rapture taking hold. Accounts of the ecstatic experience of God's presence have been part of Western monastic writings for centuries, perhaps most famously described by Teresa of Ávila, a sixteenth-century Spanish nun, who experienced the heights of physical pleasure and agony during prayer. Is this the reward for celibacy?

These Benedictines don't see it that way. 'We're not here for spiritual kicks at all,' said Father Benedict, 'We are here for hope, and through that, we get glimpses of heaven.' He explained that he is 'rather allergic' to the idea of 'experiencing' God. 'It's making God into a kind of commodity, something that's there to satisfy my needs. But that's not it at all. It's so much bigger than that. God is way, way, way beyond anything else we could describe as "experience".'

Frustratingly, from the side chapel I cannot see the statue that inspires such apparent reverie. My view of the Marian statue is partially blocked by a vast wooden candleholder on the floor in front of me, taller than I am. Its base is ornately carved with what seem to be writhing naked classical figures. I've always envied those whose faith manifests itself in direct experience of God. I've been at prayer meetings where charismatic evangelicals get swept up into speaking in tongues. Once you have seen that happen, you don't forget it. It has been described to me as a sudden change, a sense that you are not the one praying any more, but that God is praying in you, a fast and fluent song of joy and presence, a letting go. I have longed for such direct and intense religious experience, but fear it too. Perhaps for that reason, I'm still waiting.

IV

My grandmother had an old wooden dustpan with a matching curved brush to sweep the crumbs off tables after meals. She never used it, so we kids would pretend to clear up after imaginary banquets. At Pluscarden there comes a moment after dinner when the monks pass these wooden dustpans down the table. As each one finishes, he passes the brush along, wipes knife and fork on his white napkin, and stows them on a shelf beneath the table. Then he sits back and raises his hood. When all hoods are up, the meal is over.

The brush is not the only aspect of the meal that reminds me of childhood. Like most adults, I can barely remember what it feels like to be read to, but here at each meal a monk stands in a high stone pulpit to one side of the refectory and reads us a story. This tradition goes back centuries in Benedictine life, but now the texts range from biographies to books on genetics or history. Tonight, it is a biography of the late Cardinal Winning of Glasgow. It tells the story of the controversial cardinal's battles with politicians and the media. At various points, in response to funny lines, the monks smile or laugh into their napkins. The monk who reads to us has an Australian accent. His voice is hesitant, and rather flat. The whole experience is strangely comforting.

At home I read to my children, as a ritual of our own. But when I'm reading to my kids I'm close to them, hugging them, or they are climbing all over me. They interrupt and comment on the stories. Here, we sit evenly spaced along tables, and not one monk catches the eye of another. This at least enables me to indulge my habit of staring. It is like a meal for hermits, gathered in the same room. They carry the silence of their cells with them, even in these communal spaces. I like being read to, but the lack of response, the inability to thank the man who cooked our meal, the impossibility of a brief word about the snow, feels like a lack. The food is simple but good, mostly home-grown vegetables and fruit. No one asks anyone else to pass the salt.

V

There is a common room in the guest house, with a table and six chairs. Above the table hangs a single bright bulb. I've never seen that light switched off, nor the curtains drawn. It seems to burn round the clock, to offer a place of clarity, solidity, for guests who may feel the world is slipping away from them. By half past eight in the evening, the monks have retired to their cells. Tonight, despite the early starts, I cannot sleep so early, so I head for the common room. My two fellow guests are already there, sitting in the one bulb's pool of light. Talk is not small in this common room. Here, detached from the world, we discuss science and religion. In my cell that afternoon, I was reading about 'progressive detachment'.

According to this theory, evolutionary accidents have 'switched off' parts of our genome. Beavers build 'houses' out of wood, in rivers, because they are genetically determined to do so given certain environmental triggers. Human beings are not genetically driven to build shelters in this way, so we can design anything from bungalows to skyscrapers. This move away from strong instinctive connections with our environment has been termed 'detachment'. It is a kind of freedom but, according to Professor Lenny Moss, there is a downside too. It has rendered us 'sick beings' because with freedom comes a loss of stability. We cannot lose such deep attachment to ancient instincts without a sense of absence, of emptiness, of something missing.

Late at night in the wilds of Scotland, with the owls outside screeching to each other across the valley, I wonder if our 'progressive detachment', our growing freedom, was by accident or divine design? How about that for an idea – a creator God who cuts the strings of His creation to risk giving those creatures a more radical freedom? But with this freedom comes a sense of loss and sickness. And – tonight at least – sitting in the common room beneath the bulb of enlightenment, I believe the monks here may have found a way to reconnect with the source of our 'sickness', our deepest longing.

VI

At times this abbey feels like a film set – with its costume, ritual, music – and we, the guests, peering in from a side chapel, separated from the monks by a rope. At Mass each day, special effects are added by the swinging of a great metal censer. The heavy, perfumed smoke hangs at head height like a bank of fog, and blurs the lines between us. For some Protestants the use of incense is a disturbing sight, a reminder of the roots of the Mass in the theology of sacrifice.

When I left university, I worked as a documentary film-maker; during those years I saw religion at its most terrifying and its most sublime. I stood on the charred ground of Waco, Texas, where the followers of David Koresh met their own twisted apocalypse. I remember an empty sky, a dog barking miles away, and a car kicking up clouds of dust as it crossed the horizon. It felt like a place where the world could end. Christianity is inescapably bound up with sacrifice: the daily self-sacrifice of these monks as they seek to live out this tough life, and the sacrifice of self implied by the idea of 'conversion', the challenge to be 'born again'.

When I knew I was coming to Pluscarden I got back in touch with a friend I hadn't seen for a few years. He is a young man who went straight from university into a monastery, but left after a decade of monastic life. When I last saw him, he had just fled the order and was trying to rebuild his life. Now he is willing to talk, but without being named. He told me something of the price of monastic life: 'I think part of the way to the Kingdom for a monk is a profound reckoning with human aloneness – sometimes loneliness – where we face ourselves as fractured and incomplete, subject to dark (sometimes hateful) impulses as well as good and holy ones. A monk is supposed to keep to his cell and does battle there. Obviously a married Christian has to deal with this stuff as well, but I think that being celibate makes it more pressing.'

VII

I go back to my room in the middle of the day and catch my reflection in the window. The light casts my face in stark relief. I have become my grandfather. There are very few mirrors in the monastery, and without my knowing, I have aged forty years in less than a week. The monks look young for their years, but my doppelgänger in the glass looks haggard. Can silence have a physical impact? It is impossible to guess the age of the monks. I used to scoff at the idea that holiness might be visible, tangible. But some of these Benedictines seem almost translucent.

I draw the curtains, and lie down in the darkness. This silence around is deafening. It feels like a pressure, like I'm sinking too deep and will need to decompress to rise out of it. John Cage, who famously composed a silent piece of music, believed there was no such thing as true silence. There is always sound, always something. I like the idea that every time we think we have found silence there is another layer of sound beneath, like stripping off layer after layer of paint and wallpaper trying to get to the bare wall beneath. Except that there is no bare wall. It's all wallpaper and paint. Cage may be right, but if there is some sound here, some strain of deeper, richer unearthly music, I can't hear it.

When a monk visited a few days ago to see if I was settling in, my room looked like an electronics store: laptop, headphones, radio and a smartphone that couldn't get a signal. The monk was kind and said nothing about all this. But it made me feel like a lightweight, surrounded by my props. How could I confront the big void – myself – with all this kit around me? Tonight, my cell is cold and lonely, and the radio is company. I miss my wife and children, and the phone has failed me again. Its single block of network coverage slipped through the gap in the window frame and vanished into the hills. But the radio works. At minimal volume I can make out a football game. I bathe in the tinny jabber of the commentary.

VIII

'What are days for?' asked the poet Philip Larkin. Well, surely not for getting up at 4 a.m. The air is freezing. The water hurts as you rinse your face. I look down into the sink and my face shivers on the water's surface. My days at home don't start like this. They usually start with a different kind of physical jolt, as one or other of the kids jumps and climbs all over me and my wife. And now I miss it. Surely that is what days are for?

'Recalled from the shades to be a seeing being, / From absence to be on display, / Without a name or history I wake / Between my body and the day.' The longer I stay here, the more lines from Auden's *Horae Canonicae* come back to me, and the more they ring true. He associates these lines with 'Prime', the first office of daylight, a service conducted when others are sitting in cars, trains, on metros as they make their way to work. When, on my first day here, the monk told me I didn't exist, I laughed. But as the days pass, the space between my life at home and here gets wider and wider.

'Without a name or history I wake / Between my body and the day.' Auden was right. That is the chasm here, the tension. When everything that 'self' means in the world is called into question, all that remains is the space, the tension between your body and the day. The monks have no career structure, no property, no lovers and no children. I have all those things, but they mean nothing here. I think I'm losing myself. And of course, this is the point. You lose a sense of self in order to find God. 'Always let go,' Father Benedict said to me, 'never cling on. John of the Cross is fierce about this, and we strive for it, a constant letting go, to come closer to God.'

IX

Up from my desk to draw the curtains, I peer out of my window into the failing light, and watch one of the black-robed novices walk across the garden, hooded, dimly lit from the spillover of the common room's light bulb. It could be a scene from last year, or last century. Would it have looked any different seven hundred years ago? Give or take the artificial light, and the odd tree, no. I wonder if the monks learn to identify each other by their gait, their size and shape. The hooded monks are so thoroughly covered by their white or black clothes that a brother here could meet his doppelgänger and fail to recognize him.

Through the services and meals at Pluscarden I've been particularly fascinated by the novices. What have they left behind? What do they think about this life, as they lie in silence at night? And what did their families and friends make of it? 'Vocation is a very powerful, irresistible force', said Father Benedict. 'You only really do this because you have to. And it does mean that you let down parents and girlfriends. Some of us are on the brink of marriage when we come here.' I ask about the two youngest novices at Pluscarden, both in their early twenties. One has just completed a PhD in Philosophy, 'and now he's doing the laundry', says Father Benedict. The other was in the navy, working on submarines. Both are, he says, doing very well. But before they get their white robes they must serve an apprenticeship of five and a half years minimum.

Pluscarden, having gone through its lean years, now receives on average fifty serious requests a year to join the community; the majority of these requests comes from under-twenty-fives. I think about my own sons, and what I would do if one of them wanted to take up this life. I do believe that the constant prayer of these monastic communities is important, more vital than anything that goes on in the Pentagon or the UN. I like to think that I would support my sons in testing their vocation, and encourage them to follow it through if it is real. But in reality, I would be heartbroken.

x

One morning, my phone – dead for days – offers up a tiny, weak signal. I wait until 7 a.m., and call home. They are getting ready for work and school. The signal is very fragile. I don't want to raise my voice in the silence of the guest house. We establish that everyone is fine, then give up on the call. Having discovered – through the pattern of ritual, reflection and solitude – a measure of detachment, I find myself suddenly reminded of the cost of being here.

If you want to become a monk at Pluscarden, you have to commit to stability (to remain within a single community for your whole monastic life), to poverty, to obedience, plus – crucially – to celibacy. The centrality of this final vow is not just an outsider's slant. As Father Benedict told me, 'Celibacy defines us.'

The insistence of most religions (including Christianity) on self-denial as an engine of transformation has always troubled me. I'm sure this is real wisdom, but so much art and literature seems to push in the other direction, all those poems urging *carpe diem*: do it now, risk everything for more experience. But the hunger is never sated.

XI

One of my fellow guests – a Glaswegian in his sixties – sits in front of me at every service, twisted to press his back against the radiator, teeth clenched in pain. Every now and then, he traces his fingertips along a fissure in the ancient stone wall. He does this twice or three times in each service, and he stares at his fingers as he does. Is he losing concentration, distracted for a moment from the plainsong? Or is he reminding himself of the cold solid fabric of material? This is the world. This is what he stands to lose.

Losing isn't easy. Especially when the self is the subject of the loss. In 1938, broken by factory work and injured in the Spanish Civil War, the French mystic philosopher Simone Weil went on retreat to the Benedictine abbey at Solesmes. As a secular Jew and political anarchist, she did not go there to meet God. She came to recuperate, and to enjoy the aesthetic beauty of the plainsong, for which Solesmes was famous. Sitting through the daily round of offices, Weil described an effort of will, to lose herself in the beauty of the music and the building, to transcend her pain. But when she managed to let go, she got more than she bargained for. In a letter to a friend, she later described 'a presence more personal, more certain and more real than that of a human being; it was inaccessible both to sense and to imagination, and it resembled the love that irradiates the tenderest smile of somebody one loves'.

XII

This is the body. This is the moment when a round, white wafer of unleavened bread is placed on your tongue, and you swallow it. This is the most intense physical, incarnational moment of the Benedictine day. Entering the side chapel for Mass, each visitor can pick up a wafer from a silver plate by the door and place it in the chalice standing next to it. At this point, bread is bread. It means nothing. Twenty minutes later, it is God's body.

For the monks, this is the centrepiece of their life, the moment they receive the body and blood of Christ in the form of bread and wine, and they look utterly radiant as they take it, almost in tears, some of them, overwhelmed by it. Auden wrote:

You need not see what someone is doing
to know if it is his vocation,

you have only to watch his eyes:
a cook mixing a sauce, a surgeon

making a primary incision,
a clerk completing a bill of lading,

wear the same rapt expression,
forgetting themselves in a function.

How beautiful it is,
that eye-on-the-object look.

I place a wafer in the chalice, and wait for the moment when the priest walks to the side chapel. Body. This is it. And as I swallow it I am shocked again at this religion I am a part of. I do believe in the real presence in the Eucharist, and I do believe it can be – even should be – transformative. But the physicality of it, the unwillingness (in Catholic doctrine at least) to stop at symbolism or remembrance, still strikes me as astonishing and scandalous.

XIII

I fall asleep in my cell one afternoon. I wake with a jolt and cannot remember where I am. I get up quickly and open the window to hear the multiple chimes as Black Burn Glen gives way to thaw. I wonder what this routine, this lifelong all-encompassing ritual would do to me, if I lived here for years. I look out at the fields of white and remember Louis MacNeice's great poem 'Snow', and his conviction that the 'World is crazier and more of it than we think, / Incorrigibly plural.' Does the life of a monk reduce that to four grey stone walls and Latin chant? Do these Benedictines miss out on what MacNeice calls 'The drunkenness of things being various'?

Every day, as we head down the narrow track from the guest house to our side chapel, the other guests and I have had to go back for shovels to clear our path. As the thaw accelerates, more great slabs of snow drop from the guest-house roof and block the way. The more we clear it, the more seems to fall. I am powerfully drawn to this place, and have deep admiration for those who live this life. But for me, the pull of 'things being various' is too strong. As soon as I try to clear my mind, to transcend the business of living my life, I'm confronted again by the 'incorrigibly plural' world. For me, the place to encounter God is out there, amid the 'drunkenness'. As I turn the corner on to the Elgin road, a field of rooks rises, like a blizzard in reverse. Houses are appearing on the horizon. Low-lying fields display an intricate calligraphy, a record of hooves, claws and boots. The world is coming back. ■

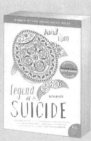

LONG DISTANCE

Victor LaValle

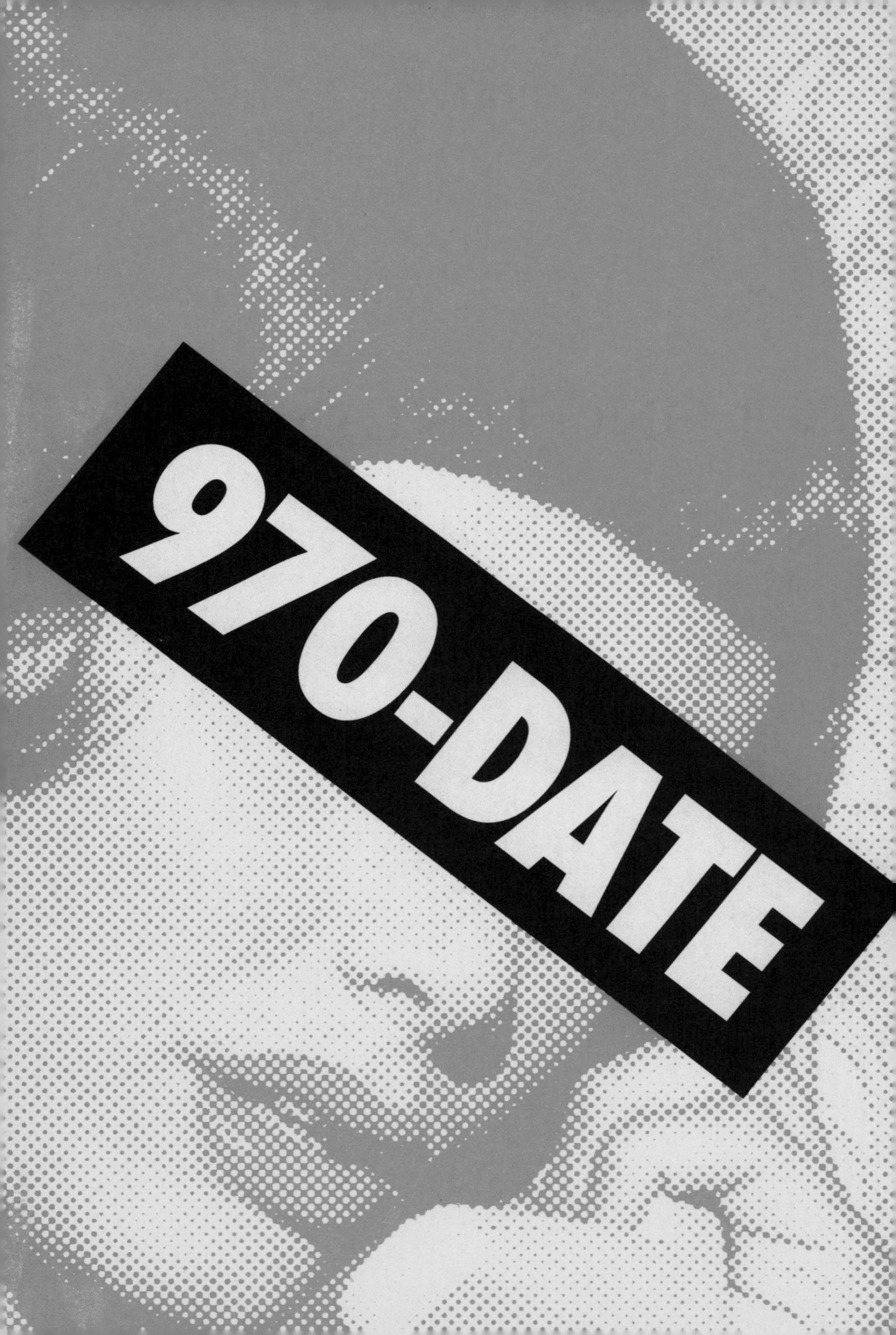
970-DATE

The most loving relationship of my early twenties cost me ninety-nine cents per minute. Her name was Margie and while I was charged to talk with her, she was not a pro. She was a fifty-year-old woman who lived in New Jersey. Two or three nights a week we called each other on a chatline. I'd dial 970-DATE and agree to have the charges billed to my telephone while Margie dialled the same number but never paid a fee. Much like at nightclubs and bars, it's a lot harder to get ladies into the room. So Margie, and the hundreds of women like her, would call the number and register as a woman, then punch through the recorded greetings from thousands of guys who were waiting to talk with them. One of those men was me.

Each guy's greeting was his name and a little something about himself. Our messages were either lewd or pornographic, nothing else. Using euphemisms about your penis counted as a true gentleman's move. I was no better than the rest. Twenty-one and horny and incapable of getting a real-world date. So instead I listened to the recorded greetings of anonymous women from all over the north-eastern United States. The women's greetings tended to differ from the men's; they spoke about amusement parks and dining out and walks on the beach. Ridiculous shit. We all knew why we were here and it wasn't to line up any dates. We were there to talk dirty into our telephones and masturbate in our separate darkened rooms. At least that was true for me and Margie.

We liked each other's voices – each other's imaginations – enough to keep calling back. We'd make appointments for the next 'meeting' and then call the line. Scroll through the many recorded messages, listening for the voice we recognized. She was Margie and I was Michael. We spent two years having phone sex and, eventually, speaking to each other off the line, but we never told each other our real names.

But why was I doing this? At twenty-one? I was in college and, in theory, surrounded by eligible women. *Besieged* by more appropriate partners. My little crew of friends enjoyed no end of sex, but my crew consisted of some sterling men. But even that's a cop-out because the schlumps and losers were actually doing all right, too, juggling a couple of women on campus. Not me though.

I was 350 pounds and didn't stand nine feet tall, so the weight didn't sit well on me. As big as a house? No. I was as big as a housing project. Lumpy and lazy; I *aspired* to lethargy. Second year of university I missed half my classes just because I couldn't pull my big butt out of bed.

But here's the thing: I was charming. Funnier than you and all your friends. Well read and well spoken. Observant and even kind. Not too easily suckered. Street-smart. In other words, I was kind of a fucking catch. And I *knew* this was true. As long as you couldn't see me. If you saw me you'd think I was the sea cow that had swallowed your catch.

Margie lived alone in the home she owned in northern New Jersey. Her daughter had grown up and married and moved away to Boston. Margie had retired because she got sick, but she'd saved her money all these years. Even leaving the workforce as young as fifty didn't give her much concern. She had enough in the bank and the mortgage had been paid off. She felt quite proud of herself, and rightly so. She never mentioned a husband, the father of her only child, and I didn't ask. During the day Margie ran errands and spent time with her neighbours. At night Margie entertained her gentleman callers.

One of them was me, Michael, a college student in upstate New York. A kid from Queens who was paying for school with a part-time job and loans. A former high-school baseball player who wanted to become a lawyer some day. I told her I looked like Derek Jeter. She said she resembled Gina Lollobrigida. Did I know who that was? The first time she told me I said, 'Of course,' and then looked the actress up.

Both our exaggerations were probably true *enough*. I did have one black parent and one white parent and I had played baseball in high school. I might as well be Derek's twin brother! As for Margie, I felt sure she was at least a woman who had brown hair. But when we finally found each other on the chatline, all suspicions fell away. She was there and I was too. Our rooms so dark we could imagine each other – and ourselves – exactly as we wanted.

'Hello, Michael.'

'Hello, Margie.'

'I missed you,' she said.

'I'm there with you now.'

'Right here in bed?'

'No. I'm outside. Looking in through your window.'

She blew out a breath. 'My neighbours will see you.'

'Then I'd better break in.'

'Aren't you afraid I'll hear you?'

I said, 'I'll hide until you're sleeping.'

'I don't keep much money in the house.'

'I don't want your money.'

'I don't have jewellery.'

'I don't want your jewels,' I said.

'Why me?' she asked.

'I saw you at the supermarket. You were wearing those tight shorts.'

'You followed me home?' she asked.

'And now I'm standing by your bed.'

Margie sighed. 'It gets so dark in here at night. I can't see anything.'

'But you can feel me getting on the bed.'

Quiet.

'Yes,' she said.

'I'm going to have to stop you from getting away though.'

She whispered, 'You could climb on my chest. Pin my arms down with your knees.'

'That would hurt you.'

'Yes,' she said.

Quiet, a little longer.

'Now open your mouth,' I said.

'I won't.'

'Don't make me smack you,' I told her.

'I'm sorry,' she said.

Even quieter now. The longest silence yet.
I said, 'If you say no to me again, I'm going to get rough.'
Margie blew into the phone softly.
'*No,*' she said.

Margie and I were 'together' for about two years. After the first year she gave me her home number and I would call at our appointed times. Neither of us expected the other to stay off the chat-lines. If I happened to hear her recorded message there, on one of our off days, calling out the name of a different man, I didn't mind. I was usually listening for a different woman. We'd defeated the madness of monogamy! It only required that we never actually see or touch each other. Sometimes we talked about me taking a bus up to her town, or her meeting me for coffee in New York City, on one of my visits home. But we never did that. And never would. Both of us knew it. She was a fifty-year-old woman with some undefined illness that forced her to retire fifteen years early. Maybe it took some toll on her physically. Maybe she was in a wheelchair, or had purple spots on her ass, I don't know. But I sure as hell never would let her see me either. If she did, how could we ever fantasize about me crouching over her chest again? In real life I'd suffocate the poor woman between my meaty thighs if we ever tried.

And yet, somehow, I convinced myself that Margie was helping to keep me tethered to the 'normal' world of relationships. I knew what we had wasn't complete, but at least we were two human beings sharing some kind of real affection. I still felt like this was infinitely better than the alternative: have you ever known men or women who don't get *any* kind of loving for years? They get *weird.* The women become either monstrously drab or they costume themselves in ways that make them seem unreal; they externalize their inner fantasies and come to believe – on some level – they really are elves or princesses or, most disturbing of all, children again. And the men? They're even worse. Men who are denied affection too long devolve into some kind of rage-filled hominoid. Their anger becomes palpable. You can almost feel the wrath emanating from their pores. Lonely women destroy themselves; lonely men threaten the world.

So with that fate in mind, I felt truly grateful for Margie. While I enjoyed phone sex with other women, Margie and I would also have real conversations after the sex was done. She'd want to know what I'd been reading in class and I'd ask about the home-improvement work she'd been doing. I enjoyed her company, her voice. And she sounded sincere when she told me she'd missed me.

So it came as a real shock when she said we'd have to stop talking.

Her daughter's husband had lost his job and their home had gone into foreclosure. The two of them, and their three-year-old child, would be moving in with Margie. There was no other way to go. Margie had plenty of space in her home. Plus she'd been so good with her money that she could afford to carry the three of them until the husband found work. And Margie wanted to do this; she loved the idea of having them close. Her only regret was that she'd have to say goodbye to me. (And to the other dudes she'd had relationships with, I gathered.) Someone would always be home and she couldn't risk the embarrassment if one of them overheard us.

So in 1995 my fifty-year-old girlfriend, the one I'd never met, broke up with me.

While she and I were 'together' I'd thought of myself like an astronaut going on one of those spacewalks outside the space shuttle. Below me I could see Earth, the glorious terrain. The place where true couples dwelled. And while I wasn't there, I could still view it. I knew what it looked like. And in time I'd make my way back into the shuttle; I'd hit the thrusters on my spaceship and return to that good soil.

But when Margie and I stopped talking it was as if the craft had blown to bits. I had plenty of oxygen in my suit, but I was no longer tethered to anything.

And the shock waves of the blast didn't send me hurtling down to Earth.

Instead, they blew me backwards.

Deeper into space.

It's funny to have to relate all this first. Because I really want to tell you about my life *after* I lost weight. What sex was like once I'd exercised and dieted myself down to 195 pounds. That's from the lifetime high of somewhere just north of 350. How did I manage the miracle? I bought a refurbished StairMaster and used it four days a week. And I joined Jenny Craig, the weight-loss system that used out-of-work celebrities in their ads. Ridiculous as it sounds, it worked.

To belabour the astronaut metaphor just a minute longer: I'd found my way back to Earth after having drifted through the lifeless void for two years. Victory parades were thrown in my honour. The President offered me heartfelt congratulations. (By which I mean my mother was incredibly proud of my change.) Here's our man, finally height and weight proportionate! Once again, a member of the human race.

But in the time I'd been away – when I'd been inhuman, I guess – I'd journeyed well past phone sex of any kind. Leapfrogged over message boards and heated Internet exchanges. I'd found another phone line where each side really did want to meet and make things happen.

I had sex – lots of it – with women who were, essentially, just like me. By which I mean more than 350 pounds *and* crippled by self-loathing. We made our introductions on the phone line, essentially negotiating the details of our affections in advance. *I want this and you want that*; *I won't do any of those things, but I will try these*. As a result I'd show up at some woman's apartment for the first time and we'd be naked in about ten minutes. Engaging in the kind of sexual fantasies that usually require six months of dating before anyone will even broach the subject. And then they probably still wait another six months before they trust each other enough actually to try it. We covered all that ground in a single night.

And I'll tell you what I learned during those two years: fat people are perverts.

By which I mean to say, loneliness perverts you.

I'm not talking about the sex. Or not exclusively, anyway. My first date as a trimmer man scared me more than my very first fist fight. Part of the reason was that I didn't even realize we were on a date.

We met each other at a party in a bar. We shook hands and exchanged a few words and then mingled among other friends. Once or twice we sat in the same frame for some of those group photos people take as a party wears on. When she sat next to me at a table and smiled before I'd said anything, I had the notion that she might be flirting with me, but the phenomenon had been so rare these last few years that I didn't trust my lying eyes. I figured my intuition had probably shrivelled up and died long ago. She wasn't flirting, she was just being friendly.

But then, a few hours into the party, she came up and asked if I liked her blouse. Her friend stood nearby, at the bar, a glass of beer in front of her mouth to try and hide the way she giggled at her friend's boldness. I was seated and she stood over me. She asked again if I liked her blouse and this time she flipped the bottom of it up and showed me her stomach.

Now *that* was flirting. Impossible to ignore. Plus, I didn't want to ignore it. This woman was beautiful by any measure. When she flipped her shirt up I saw her skin and I realized how long it had been since I'd seen a belly without stretch marks. Five years? Ten? I'm including my own in that count.

Before I left I asked if she'd go to dinner with me and when she said yes she actually went up on her tiptoes, like a kid.

I took her to a sushi restaurant and sat across from her, but after a few minutes it was clear her face showed none of the same enthusiasm as at the bar. I asked her questions about her job as a magazine editor, but she hardly answered in full sentences. I made jokes, each one worse than the last. Maybe it was just that she'd been drunk at the party. I couldn't think of an explanation for why she was acting so damn uninterested now.

Then, during another moment of silence, I looked away from her and out of the window. There were no couples between us and the store's large front windows. I saw her reflection. She was as lovely as the other night, maybe more so. She wore a sheer sweater and a skirt that flattered her long legs.

And me?

I was still wearing my coat.

Not a jacket. My *winter* coat. We'd been inside for half an hour and I hadn't taken it off. No wonder she seemed distant, even dismayed; it looked like I couldn't wait to get away.

And it wasn't just the coat. I had so many layers on. A sweater *and* a button-down shirt. And a T-shirt under them. It wouldn't have surprised me if I had thermal underwear layered down there as well. In other words, I was dressed like a fat person. We make the mistake of thinking those layers of clothing are serving to hide us. A kind of protection. Instead they only serve to make us look even bigger. Or, in this case, to make me seem like an asshole.

I wanted to explain everything to her. *I'm going through a big transition.* But I couldn't bring myself to tell her. No matter how I phrased it in my head, it always sounded like a bad pun, a sad joke. Finally, I slid my coat off, but the gesture must've seemed like pity. I popped mine off and she pulled on hers. We ate the rest of our meal quickly. I took her home on the F train but when we reached her station she said I didn't have to walk her home.

All this changed after I dated the woman with the violent boyfriend. We became friends first. We worked in the same space and at lunchtime we sometimes ate together and talked. We were attracted to each other, but did nothing about it for months. She continued to date the aforementioned bruiser and I was busy trying to live like a normal-sized man; meaning I stayed off the phone lines, I ate sensible meals, I exercised regularly, and I told no one that I'd ever been fat. The last seemed particularly important. If enough other people believed it, I hoped that I'd come to believe it too. If they treated me like a guy who'd never knocked out a dozen Krispy Kreme original glazed doughnuts in one sitting then I'd forget I ever had. I needed the outside world to convince me because I still couldn't quite believe the transformation had been real.

So all of the fall of 1998, I'm flirting with this woman but keeping a respectful distance. Getting closer and then pulling away. And she was doing the same. This slow build felt exciting and frustrating. But each time I saw her again my feelings seemed even stronger. And that was a shock too. *Feelings*. Not to be too self-pitying (or self-aggrandizing), but I hadn't really cared about a woman outside my family since Margie and I hung up our phones in 1995.

Christmas, 1998. A little bit of partying. A lot of alcohol. I remember the first time she put her arms around me, outside a bar. I held my breath as she clasped her hands around my waist; then she rested her head against my chest.

And finally the two of us are stumbling back to her building. We climb the stairs to her apartment. Open the front door, listen for her room-mate, and when it seems we're alone we fall across her living-room couch. I'm on my back and she's on top of me. She undoes my jeans and slides them down and lifts her skirt. She climbs back on top of me.

And as much as I'm enjoying myself, as I anticipate the next step with three years' worth of pent-up glee, I'm also not really there. As soon as my pants slide down to my knees and my shirt rides up above my belly I feel myself wince, as if preparing for an explosion. And I realize I've been thinking of my clothes as if they were the casing around a live bomb.

Have you ever had out-of-body sex? It's not the same as that tantric business. As soon as my skin touched open air my mind drifted away. I watched myself and this woman having some wonderfully energetic sex. I even felt proud of the guy down there because he seemed so free. *He* was laughing and gripping her hips, but *I* was floating up by the ceiling. That body and the person inside it weren't connected to each other. While the body worked up a sweat, I remained cool on the outside, keeping watch; I felt sure that if this woman saw me at the wrong angle, or in the wrong light, her lust would suddenly fold up and be packed away.

Then she reached down and touched my stomach; I'd lost a lot of weight but the skin there was a little loose, and there were faint stretch marks along the bottom that looked like dried-out riverbeds. She put her hand on my stomach and I sucked my belly in. Understand, I didn't even have that belly anymore but that didn't make the belly any less real to me.

Her hand stayed there on my stomach and I waited to hear her say, 'Stop.' Or, 'Get off me.' Or a groan of disgust.

But instead she did the most perfect thing. For which I remain grateful.

She lifted her hand and then brought it back down hard. She smacked me.

But not out of revulsion; not to punish me.

She looked down at me and gritted her teeth.

'*Harder*,' is the only thing she said.

Later that night the violent boyfriend showed up. We were in her bedroom by now, zonked out from sex and bourbon, when the sound of the building's buzzer woke us up. In my tired mind it was the sound of a wasp, a swarm of wasps, and I woke up swatting at the air. Finally, I realized someone was downstairs, in the lobby, trying to get in.

'It's him,' she said quietly.

'How do you know it's not your room-mate?'

'My room-mate doesn't ring the bell. My room-mate has the keys.'

Now we both sat up and listened as the buzzing continued. I'd met the boyfriend before, when he'd visited her at work. Not intimidating. The guy reminded me of Jean-Paul Sartre, actually, owlish like that. After he'd left she'd told me about how violent he could get and I thought she was making a confession about her own abuse. But it wasn't like that. He'd never swung on her. Or even used a cross word. But she swore she'd watched him chop down guys the size of redwood trees. You can't always guess that kind of thing, just from looking.

I slid out of bed and said, 'I'll go talk to him.'

But she frowned. 'You really don't want to do that.'

I thought of her stories about him. I was *much* smaller than a redwood now.

I slid back next to her and we lay there as he continued zapping the buzzer. We wondered if her room-mate would show up and let him in. Caught sleeping in bed with another man's woman: that's a surefire way to get your ass snuffed. She fell asleep long before I did. I spent hours lying there, alert.

By dawn I still hadn't gone to sleep, but I had stopped worrying over the violent boyfriend long ago. I lifted my hand until it was bathed in the morning light coming through the thin curtains. I still couldn't believe what I saw. My new hand, slim enough to show the wrist bones; the knuckles no longer lost in flesh. But this hand hadn't replaced the old one; instead it was like this hand had grown *around* the fatter one somehow. Both were there but only one could be seen. ■

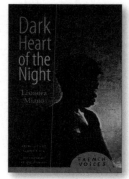

THE BLUE ZOO

Chris Offutt

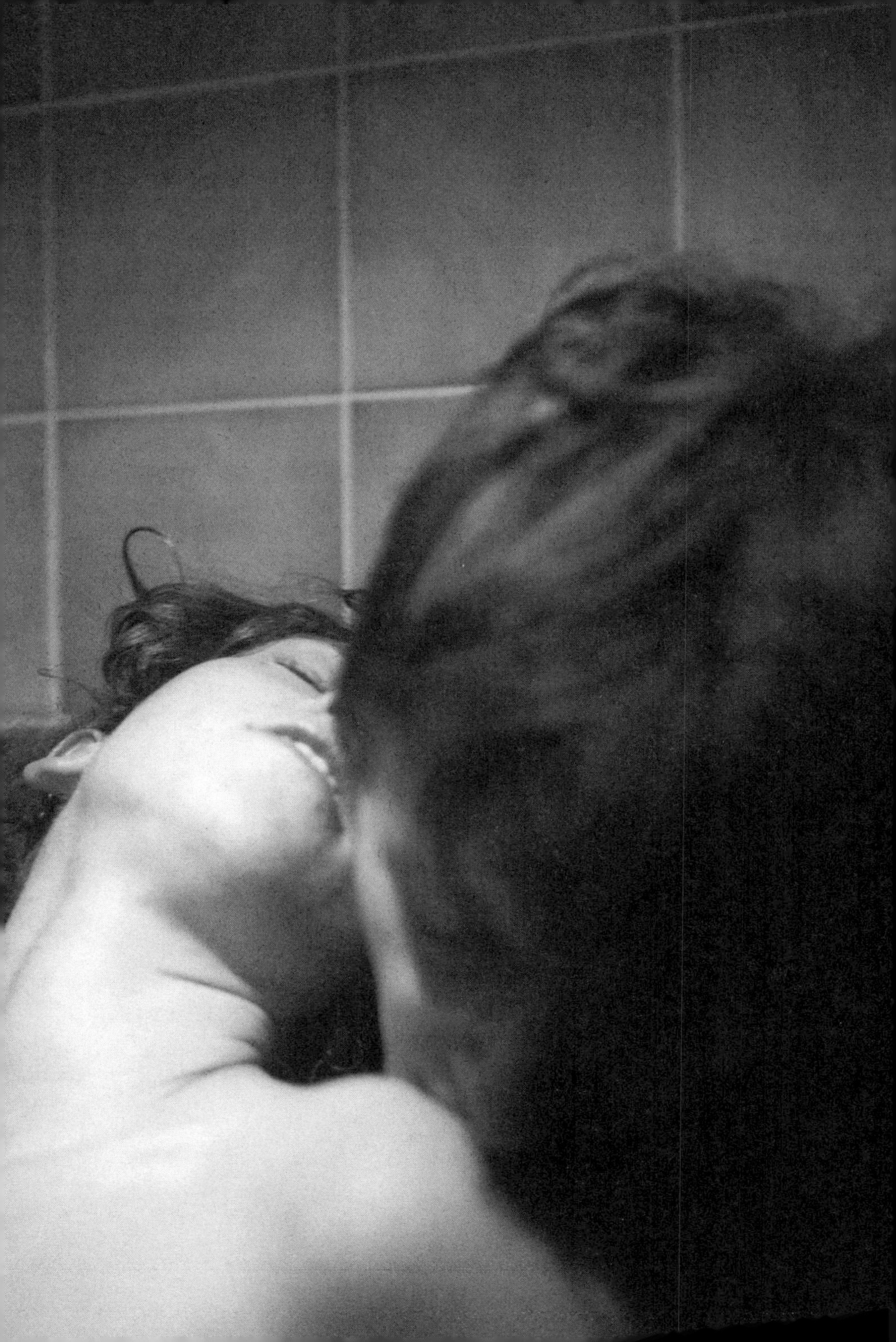

Cecil found work at the lumber yard in Rocksalt and moved into the county's biggest trailer court. More people lived there than in his home hollow, and he considered it the next best thing to town. His trailer matched all the rest – a blue exterior, louvred windows and spindly steps to the aluminum door. Next door was a drive-in movie theatre, its screen mangled by weather. Steel posts held detachable speakers that clipped to the window of each car. Cecil could see the screen from his bedroom window.

The Blue Zoo was practically swimming with women, and Cecil believed smoking marijuana in his yard sent a message that he was ready to party with the ladies. So far he'd only met men, but Cecil had faith that word would circulate and a slew of divorcees would soon be knocking on his dented blue door. They were the ones to go for.

Cecil's notions about sex were based on the bragging of equally inexperienced friends, a crumbling copy of a porn magazine, observation of pets and misguided imaginings in general. The process seemed fraught with the likelihood of error and embarrassment, even pain. As a child he'd decided he would never marry because the bride and groom kissed each other in public, and he knew he could never do that. But now, at nineteen, he'd matured. He had his own place, drove his own car and was letting his hair grow. Twice in the last week he'd seen the same girl walking alone at the edge of town. He slowed but didn't stop; wanting to make sure she heard the rumble of his Impala. If he saw her again, Cecil resolved to talk with her.

Lucy lived alone with her grandfather who, reticent in general, was silent as a grave about the body. When she got her period in fifth grade, she hid in the bathroom until a teacher drove her home. The woman spoke privately with Lucy's grandfather, whose only reaction was a gradual reddening of the face that steadily increased until the teacher began to wonder how human skin could produce such a deep hue of crimson. Maybe the old man had a little Shawnee in him. He refused her assistance in the way the teacher recognized, a country pride that hid his own fear.

Within a week, the preacher's wife visited the house, invited in an oblique fashion by Lucy's grandfather having mentioned the need to a neighbour man who told his wife, whose cousin attended church. The preacher's wife arrived, nervous as a long-tailed cat in a room full of rocking chairs. Her husband waited in the car. Lucy's grandfather stood outside and the men nodded to each other across the dusky yard but didn't speak, each feeling pastured away from women's business. The preacher's wife laid out the facts as best she understood them, then gave Lucy a penny for birth control. In the company of men, Lucy was to hold the penny tight between her knees and never let it fall. For now, Lucy should take aspirin and lie in bed until her monthlies went away. It was an unclean time, and Lucy was to read the Bible, avoid handling raw meat or standing in direct moonlight.

The preacher's wife spoke for a good half-hour and left, pleased with her service to the hapless young girl. She joined her husband and they drove in silence, leaving the dark hollow's dirt road for one of packed creek rock, and finally easing on to the narrow blacktop. The preacher remarked that he didn't know which was worse at night – going up the hollers or out the ridges. His wife said nothing, aware only of her own thwarted desires of youth, craving passion, tenderness and bliss. She put her feelings away like a folded note. There was no solution but prayer.

Lucy gave the penny to her grandfather because it was the old-time kind with two stalks of wheat on the back. He refused to look at her and she went to bed. He listened to the rasp of locusts fade in the darkness. He was over his head in every way, a short dog in tall grass. The mysteries of women were foreign but he knew the ways of men. He squeezed the penny tight. He'd beat the holy hell out of any boy who came sniffing around the house.

Over the next few years, Lucy learned to accommodate her body's betrayal, and at the eighth-grade sock hop she kissed a boy who wanted to kiss her again. When she refused, he told his buddies that she put out like a Coke machine. She spent the first two years of high school fending off a reputation she didn't know existed.

In the spring of her junior year, Lucy missed the bus and faced a fourteen-mile walk home. It had happened twice the week before and she'd gotten a ride with a neighbour lady who worked in town. This time a car slowed and she didn't recognize the boy driving so she ignored him. He circled back and she accepted a ride, but kept her hand on the door handle. He drove her to the foot of her hollow, where they sat in the car and talked for half an hour. She agreed to meet him again, but only if he swore never to visit her house.

Lucy's sudden cheer surprised her grandfather and made him momentarily grateful before his thoughts returned to the more promising past. In the last few years, drinking had latched to him like a leech. After World War II he had taken a stand in the hollow and now he felt like he'd driven his ducks to a dry puddle – the death of his wife, his daughter and his son-in-law, a grandson off in Texas building houses, and now little Lucy not so little. He noticed the changes in her body and hated himself for it.

At night he sat in the woods beyond the house pouring whiskey in his head and thinking of his own boyhood during the Depression. His family had relied on his sharp sight for bringing in game. They ate the squirrels to death, then worked their way through rabbit, deer, possum, groundhog, beaver and bear. Only the skunks had flourished in safety. During the forties all the animals returned, as he had after D-Day. Sometimes he wished he'd died on Omaha Beach. He was shot twice but kept stumbling forward, and now felt stuck with life. He sipped whiskey. Starlight streamed among the trees. He missed his wife. He drank more whiskey. Rain came. Instead of going inside, he found shelter beneath the canopy of overlapping limbs, sitting on a stump in the dark fog that blotted trees and foiled the hunting of owls that couldn't see their own wingtips.

He capped the bottle. Brush rustled, the damp leaves muffling an animal's approach. The tapered face of a bewildered doe appeared in the night's thick air. He clubbed the deer across the head with the bottle, spraying the ground with shattered glass. The stunned doe stood blinking. He shoved the jagged edge into the doe's neck, twisted his wrist, and stabbed again with a ferocity born of combat. The deer kicked a single foreleg without any understanding of what had just occurred, aware only of the sudden blow, the pain, and now the weakness. It crumpled to the ground and the night continued as if nothing important had happened.

Lucy let Cecil do anything he pleased with her for no other reason than it felt good to be wanted. She mistook his clumsy trepidation for respect. He liked her, she could tell, and she liked his life. His trailer was new, much nicer than her house, with an electric fan and a colour TV. Lucy loved the day-long anticipation of seeing him after school. She loved the new sense of her body, as if it was a grove hidden in the hills recently exposed to light. She loved deceiving her grandfather, who never asked where she was or who she was with. Lucy supposed that she loved Cecil as well. After all, he kept his face shaved for her and chewed a twig of sassafras to flavour his mouth. Cecil was everything she'd ever lacked – friend, lover, sibling, parent. She felt released from a confinement she hadn't known existed.

At dusk they sat on the steps of Cecil's trailer, waiting for the drive-in movie to start. Cecil showed her how to smoke pot by punching a hole in a pop can and using it as a pipe. Lucy loved that he knew things like that.

'We'll be together forever,' she said.

'Maybe we can open a little store.'

'We'll be old together.'

'We'll die at the exact same moment.'

'We'll be buried in the same grave.'

'Our bones will stay together.'

'For longer than we were alive.'

Cecil turned the sound up on his television and they watched the drive-in movie, laughing when the TV dialogue conflicted with the action on the giant screen.

School ended in spring with rainwater engraving gullies down the hillsides. Morning sun burned the dew to drifting strands of mist. They drove dirt roads that linked the ridges like ribbons woven through a sweater. Twice they ran the car battery down listening to the radio and had to push-start it. The cicadas roared like waterfalls around them. She turned seventeen and he gave her a lace handkerchief that she kept in her sleeve.

By August, Lucy's monthlies had stopped, her body ached and she began her days with nausea. She didn't bother attending school. She avoided Cecil, and knew she couldn't talk to her grandfather. The only option was to follow a trail deep in the woods to the farthest ridge. Lucy didn't know if the old woman was myth or fact, living or dead, but Lucy had always heard about her.

She set out in September amid a flurry of leaves swirling from the trees. Autumn was arriving early. The sky hung above the hills like a bolt of fresh-dyed fabric. The air cooled as she climbed the faint path. Squirrels watched her from the boughs of walnut. The maples were scarlet, the poplars bare, only the oaks still lingering green. A bobcat sniffed her passage and went the opposite way. Trees grew farther apart, separated by fern and rock. Lucy smelled smoke. The faint path opened to a field clouded by a gauze of milkweed's silky seeds shifting in the breeze. A small house sat with the mountain at its back.

Pearl had known since dawn that someone was coming. She stoked her fire with quick-burning cedar, certain the sweet scent would draw the girl. They came day and night, but today was the first in more than twenty years. Pearl supposed word was out that she was dead. The girl emerged from the woods and Pearl studied the carriage of her back and hips as she crossed the pillow field, though Pearl had not made a milkweed pillow for many years. There was a wildness to the girl, a fierce strength, but that was always true for those who came. She opened the door as the girl trod upon the oak-plank porch.

Lucy moved to a chair. The woman used a gourd to dip water from a wooden bucket. Lucy found it easy to talk to this ancient stranger whose face was lined like clay dirt in a drought, crevices linked by tiny cracks. Her skin was earth itself.

Pearl listened less to the girl than the heart behind the language, the story washing over her like a light rain blown through a screen door. There was the familiarity of despair. Then Pearl ran her hands along the girl's belly, and prodded with two fingers, measuring the tautness of skin, gauging the parcel within.

'Can you help me?' the girl said.

And there it was, the words between them like a swaying bridge, the same reason all the girls came to her. At one time they brought gifts, supplying a ritual of exchange that broke a trail for discussion. This girl was direct, there'd be no dallying about. She was young and lustrous, surprisingly unafraid. She was also four and a half months pregnant, too far along for Pearl to administer a herbal potion to induce miscarriage. Pearl suggested talking to the father, but understood the futility; the boy would go his own way as they always did.

'You can stay here,' Pearl said, 'if you're wanting to.'

The girl shook her head and left the house and crossed the field. Pearl watched the woods until full dark drained along the land beneath a dazzle of stars. She hadn't seen anyone in four years and didn't want another visit. She woke up tired no matter how long she slept. She couldn't hear well. Her memory was an apron that had lost its pockets, carrying only their faded imprint. Soon the snow would fly. Her bones were cold and the flesh impossible to warm. She was no longer needed. The first night of hard frost, Pearl resolved to lie in the deepest hollow and wait for oblivion to relieve her of her burdens.

With the pregnancy confirmed, Lucy no longer feared it. She would marry Cecil. Her grandfather would box in the porch for an extra room and her brother would come home from out West. The sounds of night rose around her and the air turned cold as a creek rock. Fallen leaves covered the path. She headed vaguely north, but landmarks were foreign and the route twisted with geography. She decided to look ahead and figure where the trail didn't lead, then go whichever direction was left. Lucy arrived home long past midnight, her grandfather already deep in his whiskey slumber. She drifted to sleep feeling like a grown-up.

In the morning Lucy tidied the house and made coffee for her grandfather. He poured a second cup. She told him she was pregnant. He uttered one word: 'Whore', and struck her across the face, snapping her head sideways. He went outside and climbed the hill to a spot he favoured for the view of the next hill, and sat in awe at his own rage.

Lucy took a sweater and left. The hollow was still cold, but the dirt road ended at the sunny blacktop. The first car stopped, a man driving his mother to the grocery in town. He asked if she was in school and Lucy told him she was seventeen, and the man nodded politely and said he'd quit school at sixteen himself. His mother said she didn't make it past the fourth grade and it hadn't hurt her any. They dropped Lucy at the Blue Zoo. The drive-in lot was cluttered with trash, abandoned chairs and even a sagging tent. Empty beer cans glittered in the sun.

Cecil was at work, and his absence made the trailer empty and lifeless. She washed the dishes and straightened the rooms. She figured they'd put the baby at the trailer's end, furthest from the movie screen. She lay in bed, hoping not to wrinkle the sheets she'd pulled taut. She wanted their home to be perfect when Cecil heard her news.

Cecil hadn't seen Lucy in nearly three weeks. He'd dutifully stayed away from her house, but he missed her smile and quiet laugh. He worried that she'd met someone else, or that he'd made her mad somehow. Worse, the drive-in had booked a series of X-rated movies for the final month of the season. People who lived in the Blue Zoo moved lawn chairs on top of their trailers. A man began selling beer from the back of a truck. Music from car stereos carried across the drive-in lot, drowning the movie sound, but no one cared because giant naked people were gyrating against the glorious backdrop of the autumn hills. Within a week, the drive-in had transformed to a grand party that ran half the night. Church people slowly cruised by to confirm the evidence of sin, then passed again to double-check. There were so many wrecks that a tow-truck operator parked nearby. Cecil wanted to see the sex movies with her, then try some of the more complicated manoeuvres.

He drove home from work disconsolate, unsure what to do. Sawdust coated his clothes and his fingers contained tiny splinters of wood. Lucy met him at the trailer door. They clung to each other at the top of his rusted metal steps, the screen door banging in the breeze, the vast future ahead like a supple lane winding through an orchard in perpetual blossom. She told him she was pregnant.

His initial disbelief faded as he understood there was no reason for Lucy to lie, and it wasn't the sort of thing she'd be mistaken about. Though terrified, he didn't mind – it made him more of a man. Cecil told her he would marry her. A wife. A child. A family. Then, suddenly, he didn't think he could do it. Then he knew he had to. He opened a pint of whiskey to celebrate. Lucy refused, thinking of the baby, and he knew she'd make a good mother.

At dusk they sat outside on a blanket with their backs against the tin metal skirt that ran along the bottom of the trailer. They watched the drive-in screen until the first sexual episode – nothing fancy but exciting nonetheless, embarrassing even, and both felt grateful for the darkness. Fog was drifting down the hollow. People left their cars and moved closer to the screen, cheering the close-ups. Someone built a bonfire. The temperature began to drop and Lucy blew into her hands for warmth. They went in the trailer and undressed and she didn't complain when he stretched from the bed to peer through the window at the movie screen. Lucy slid into the sleep of exhaustion, grateful and happy. Cecil rose silently and tucked the blankets beneath her chin. She didn't look pregnant, just fuller, like an apple tree laden with fruit, the boughs adding more gravity to the trunk.

Sex hadn't been quite what he'd imagined. Lucy was as enthusiastic as ever, but the woman on the screen had screamed and thrashed without a trace of shyness. He wanted to marry the actress instead of Lucy.

Cecil was suddenly sober. He'd had sex with one girl and didn't want her to be the only one for ever, which would be the case if he got married. His uncles and cousins were in that situation. They kept dogs and guns, drank beer in the garage, and worked on cars with their buddies. Their wives cooked and cared for kids, banding together with other women as if men were a common foe. Each couple gained weight slowly until they were two fat strangers sharing quarters, locked into ingrained habits of defiance, compliance and television.

Cecil quietly put his TV in the car's back seat. He slid open the drawers to his bureau and removed the few clothes he owned and stuffed them into a paper bag. No one in Cecil's family had ever believed in banks, but he was too smart to hide cash beneath the mattress. He had $350 in an envelope concealed at the bottom of a bag of flour. He kept forty and left the rest on the table. With a toothbrush in his pocket he was packed. In a final act of generosity, he hauled the television back inside and set it on the table beside the money. The air was very cold. He got his car started on the third try and drove it a few trailers away, where he stopped to let the engine warm. He smoked a cigarette. It never occurred to him that he would revisit this decision for the rest of his life.

That night the temperature dropped sixty-two degrees in six hours; a state record. A lack of heat forced the projectionist from the booth before changing the last reel, and the raucous party moved inside various trailers until the liquor ran out. The following morning was a Saturday and few people were about. A heavy layer of frost covered the ground. There had been a dusting of snow but wind moved it, leaving patches of white against the brown earth. The sky lay flat and blue between the hills. A man driving home from the store saw a stray dog shivering in the drive-in lot. He went home, drank his coffee, became concerned about the dog and went outside to give it a biscuit. The dog was behaving oddly, moaning low in its throat, walking a circle, staying near something mounded on the ground. The man focused all his animal-calming abilities on the dog and didn't notice the dead woman until the dog licked her hand. He ran to his trailer and called the sheriff. Within half an hour all but the most diligent of Blue Zoo sleepers had been awakened by the sirens from various emergency vehicles.

The young woman's body lay along a vague boundary that defined the town limits. Rocksalt police claimed the county was responsible, and the county sheriff said it was town jurisdiction. The cops argued all morning. They finally agreed to call the state police, a last resort, because they hated giving anything to the Smokies. The trooper arrived with his air of superiority and radioed headquarters, requesting a county surveyor to solve the problem. Someone threw a blanket over the body. The dog dragged it away.

Lucy woke in a languorous fashion, enjoying the warmth of the bed. She'd never stayed overnight with Cecil and when she reached for him, she was surprised that his side of the bed was empty. She dressed and wrapped a quilt around her shoulders. She saw the TV first, then the money. Boot prints stencilled in flour led to the door. His car was gone. Dazed and numb, Lucy joined the people surrounding the body of the young woman. A deputy kicked the dog and it cowered near Lucy at the back of the crowd. The surveyor ascertained that the body lay within the Rocksalt city boundary by four feet. The county coroner pronounced the woman dead and speculated that it was from exposure. Paramedics carried a stretcher to the body. They strained to lift it, but the woman was frozen to the ground.

The chief of police assumed control. He didn't want the state trooper taking over again, and he wanted to show the county sheriff how things ought to work. He dispatched a man for a propane torch and upon his return, the chief lit the torch and applied heat to the hard ground. The flame shook until he got over his nerves and settled into the job of softening the earth. A thin line of smoke lifted from the body, followed by the smell. The chief stood quickly, struggling not to gag. The crowd thinned by half but many people still watched closely, including Lucy, her head covered by a blanket that carried the scent of Cecil's aftershave. Beside her, the dog trembled and moaned.

The chief heated the earth around the body while another man removed the thawed dirt with a shovel. He dug at a slant, angling beneath the woman's remains until the body rested on a shelf of frozen dirt, held by a central column. The chief broke the column and the platter of earth fell sideways. Four men lifted the body cupped in dirt, and carried it to the ambulance. The authorities nodded respectfully to each other as if they'd enjoyed full cooperation, and drove away. One by one, people returned to the warm safety of their trailers.

Lucy stood alone in the empty lot strewn with garbage. The dead woman hadn't been much older than her. The dog circled the hole, sniffing the earth. A jet streamer bisected the space between the hills, its white contrail fading into the flannel sky. The plane was filled with people going somewhere, leaving one life for another. Lucy realized she would have to do that too.

The dead woman turned out to be from Carter County, which didn't surprise anyone. Her blood was filled with alcohol and a drug called Quaalude, which turned out to be the dog's name, inscribed on its collar. Her brothers spent three days in Rocksalt looking for revenge. They were rough boys without much luck, and wound up in jail for beating on an old retarded man.

The Blue Zoo's reputation transcended the county and it became known as the wildest place to live in the hills. The drive-in closed. Kids broke the windows out of the snack bar, and weeds grew in the rutted field. The projection screen stood like a giant tombstone. Lucy gave birth in late winter.

No one remembered the dead girl's name. ■

GRANTA

ROSELAND

Rebecca Lenkiewicz

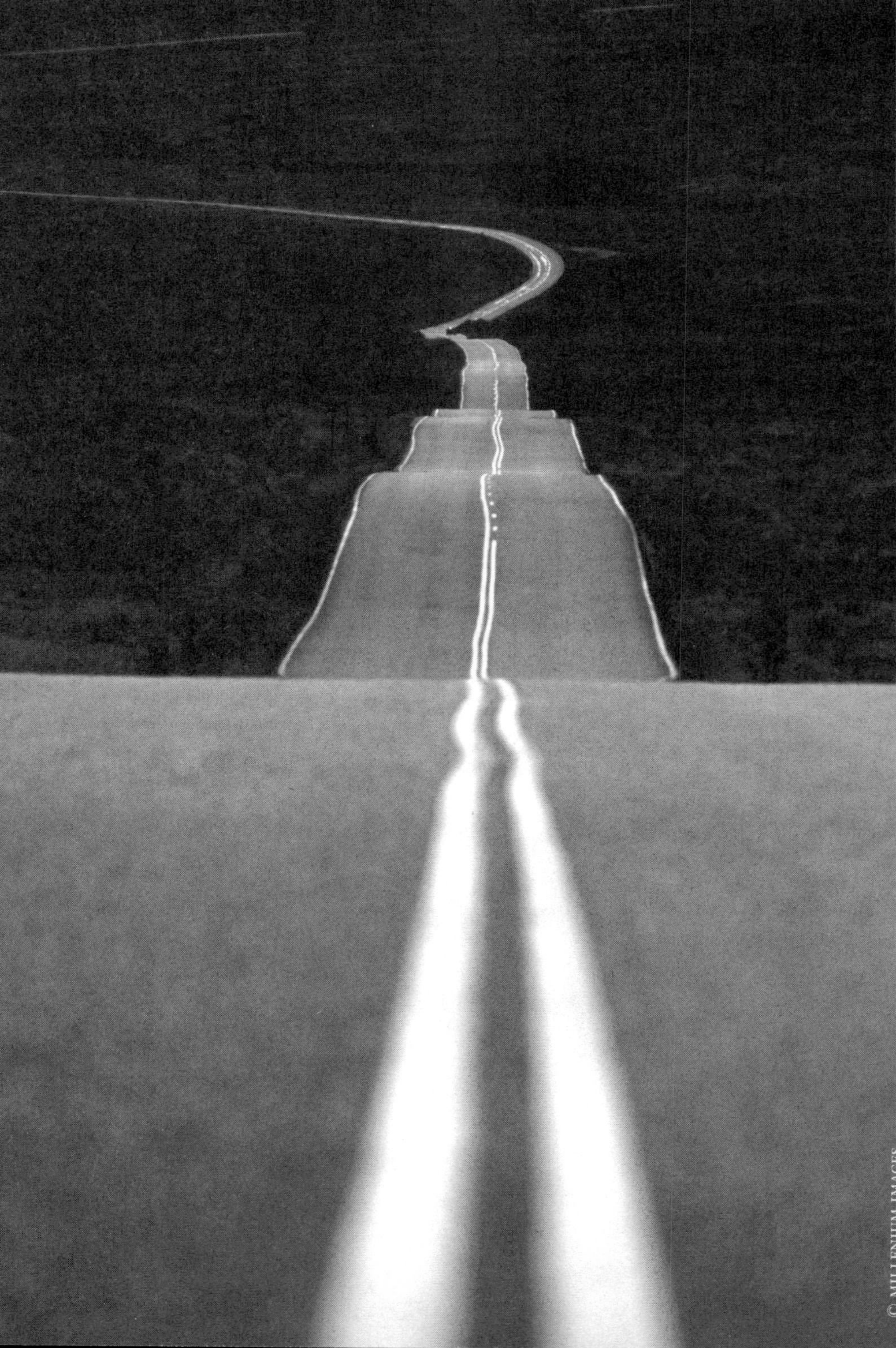

I'm twenty-one. On a Greyhound bus going from New York to San Francisco. I haven't planned a route. I simply head west and take my time. I sleep on the buses at night or at an occasional hostel. I have been on the road for weeks and the loneliness is palpable. But America's landscape fills me. I live on pretzels and bagels, and bus stations start to feel a little like home. I cry at the beauty of the Grand Canyon. The electric-blue birds that fly from the bottom of the gash to the top. The crazy goats. I decide I could die happy on the Angel Trail sometime when I'm old as the light changes with the sun going down. I become caught by the rhythm of travelling through darkness. The anonymity of it appeals to me. Attention from men is routine simply because I am young and alone.

A Vietnam veteran sits next to me and starts to tell me his story. At one point in his narrative it becomes essential for him to hold his head in his hands and throw his face towards my crotch, his hooch breath hot and regular into my jeans. He does not move or continue his story. I don't stop him from breathing heavily into my pubis bone. He clutches at my sacrum. It's a silent plea. 'Can I stay here? Back where it all began?' I stare at the top of his head and out of the window. Then I stroke his hair, and feel strangely alive and maternal. A second veteran confesses all to me a week later and curls up identically into my lap, crying. I offer no comfort this time, suspicious that word has gone around on pirate walkie-talkies about a gullible gal.

The bus drives towards Texas. It's 2 a.m. I watch the highway and its lights. I'm sat next to a plump boy in dungarees. He has dark curly hair and is most likely a twenty-year-old virgin. I fall asleep against his shoulder. Half waking I feel the warmth of his arm. I put my coat over me like a blanket. In doing so I have created a hidden place. Soon I feel his hand brush against my knee testing my depth of sleep. I fake a dream, a light sigh. He places his hand tentatively upon my leg. Then it moves to my thigh. I edge nearer to him, still faking, complicit. His hand travels an inch higher every ten minutes. He ends up exploring me with his young fingers. I feel his hydraulic bliss of being allowed in. I don't feel pleasure. Or pain. My isolation subsides, replaced by his need. And that is enough to allow him to continue. It's a game. An act that I want to be good at. I finally tire of it and turn away from him as though the dream bed has shifted again. He holds me gently for miles, my back to him. Through one state and into another.

I pretend to wake and the boy in dungarees stares at me. He puts his hands in his pockets. The sky is powder blue and the bus smells of disinfectant and petrol. 'Morning,' he says. He is more direct than I had expected. I smile. 'The next stop is Roseland,' he says, unabashed. 'I live in Roseland. Would you want to get off there?' I am probably a year older than him yet I feel like Mother Time compared to his boyishness. 'Would you?' he repeats. And I shake my head, silently saying goodbye to a life of white fences. And apples. And rosy-cheeked children in dungarees. Or maybe just an alcoholic existence at a gas station. ■

GRANTA

THIS IS FOR YOU

Emmanuel Carrère

TRANSLATED BY LINDA COVERDALE

Pour certains écrivains, c'est la
même chose : nul point n'est
jamais final. Mais il arrive aussi que
ce soit l'œuvre elle-même – par sa
structure ou son parti pris technique – qui impose cette forme sans
fin. Exemple : le deuxième roman
d'Adam Thirlwell, L'Évasion. « En
l'écrivant, j'avais dans la tête une
image de spirale », explique ce
jeune écrivain britannique, l'un
des plus talentueux de sa généra-
tion, dont les Éditions de l'Olivier

An editor at *Le Monde* calls to invite me to write a short story for their summer series. These are supplements that appear on the weekends and enjoy a significant readership, it seems. Seven or eight thousand words on the subject of travel. My first impulse is to refuse, because I can't come up with an idea, and then I remember that Sophie had once asked me: Why don't you write an erotic story? For me. I'd said: I'll think about it. And I do think about it. In fact, I call the journalist back to say that I'll take him up on his offer after all, but under one condition, which is that I can choose the date of publication. That can be arranged, he says. So, great. It's the end of May, and I want the piece to appear in *Le Monde* as a surprise for Sophie on 20 July, when she will be taking the train to join me and my family on the Île de Ré. I polish off the story in three days, just before leaving for Kotelnich. I don't tell Sophie anything about my plan. I have no idea that this story will horribly damage my life, and I don't think I have ever written anything with such ease and delight. I'm not brooding over my grandfather any more. I'm having fun, laughing out loud, quite pleased with myself.

At the station news-stand, before getting on the train, you bought *Le Monde*. Today is the day my story is being published, I told you this morning on the phone, adding that it would make excellent reading for your trip. You said three hours was a lot to fill with one story, and you'd be taking along a book as well. To avoid making you suspicious, I agreed that yes, that would probably be wise, but now I'll bet you that whatever book you chose, you won't be opening it.

You took your seat, watched other people settle in; there are probably quite a few passengers. Someone must have been sitting next to you: man or woman; young or old; pleasant or not; I don't know. With plenty of time to kill, you waited until the train pulled out to pick up the newspaper. Graffiti-covered walls along the railway tracks, the route south, the exit from Paris. You skimmed the first page, and the last one, which has the profile of me. Then you took the special insert section, opened it, refolded it; I hope nothing in the story caught your eye in the meantime … And you began to read.

Strange feeling, no?

What's strange, first of all, is that you know nothing about the story. We were together when I wrote it, but I didn't want to show it to you. I told you evasively that it was more or less science fiction. At first glance, it's rather reminiscent of that novel by Michel Butor, *La Modification*, which takes place on a train and is written in the second person. I suppose that some readers who've reached this point have already thought of that. But you, you're too astonished to think of Michel Butor. You are realizing that instead of a story, I have written you a letter that 600,000 people – that's the circulation of *Le Monde* – have been invited to read over your shoulder. You're touched, perhaps a trifle uneasy too. You wonder what I have in mind.

I have a proposition for you. From this moment on, you will do everything I tell you to do. To the letter. Step by step. If I tell you, stop reading at the end of this sentence and don't start again for ten minutes, you'll stop reading at the end of this sentence and not start again for ten minutes. That's just an example, it doesn't count. But the general idea – you'll go along with it? You'll trust me?

Well now, I'm telling you: at the end of this sentence, stop reading, close the section, and spend precisely ten minutes asking yourself what I have in mind.

You other readers – gentlemen and ladies (in particular) whom I do not know – I have no right to tell you what to do, but I urge you to play along.

There. Ten minutes have passed.

Everyone else, I don't know about them, but you, you must have figured it out.

I would now like you to make an effort and concentrate. A modest effort, though, because I'll be asking a lot more of you later on, and easy does it. Simply try to visualize yourself. First, your immediate surroundings, many variables of which escape me: are you facing forwards or backwards? Next to the window or aisle? On a single banquette or one facing other passengers (clearly an important detail)? And now you, seated, with the special section open on your lap. Do you want me to describe you, to help you out? Actually no, I don't believe that's necessary, first because I'm not very good at description, and also because the idea is not only to make you – *you* – get wet with excitement, but to make every other woman reading this get wet as well, and too precise a description of you would put them off. Even just saying a tall blonde with a long neck, slender waist and ample hips, that's already too much. So I won't say anything like that. Same ambiguity regarding your clothes. I would obviously prefer a summery dress, bare arms and legs, but I was careful not to make any such suggestion, and you may well be wearing trousers, practical for travelling – we can handle that. However many layers you've put on – and in this season it's reasonable to hope there is just one – the only sure thing is that underneath you are naked. I remember a novel in which the narrator realizes with a sense of wonder that at all times women are naked under their clothes. I shared, I still share, that wonderment. I would like you to think about that for a while.

Now, the second exercise: to become conscious of the fact that you are naked under your clothes. Focus on, first, those areas of skin in direct contact with the air – face, neck, hands, plus parts of your arms and legs; second, the areas covered with fabric, and here a whole host of nuance comes into play, depending on whether the cloth clings (undergarments, tight jeans) or hangs more or less loosely (blouse, calf-length skirt). There's still a third part, which I've kept for last: all areas of skin in contact with other areas of skin – for example, beneath that same skirt, a pair of crossed thighs, the underside of one resting on top of the other, the upper calf against the side of the knee. Close your eyes and take inventory of all the points of contact: your skin with the air, with fabric, with a different area of skin, or with yet something else (your forearms on the armrest, your ankle against the plastic of the seat in front of you). Review whatever your skin touches, whatever touches your skin. Itemize everything that's happening on the surface of *you*.

Fifteen minutes.

There's a moment that is always delicate – pleasurable, but delicate – during phone sex, and it's the moment when one shifts from normal dialogue to the heart of the matter. Almost invariably this begins with asking the other person to describe her position in space ('Mmmm, I'm on my bed …'), then the clothing in question ('Just a T-shirt, why?'). Next comes the request to slip a finger in somewhere between clothing and skin. Now here, I hesitate. It's like chess or psychoanalysis, where it seems that everything depends on the first move. The classic target would be a breast, to be approached in various ways, depending on whether or not it is encased in a bra. Usually, you wear one. I know most of them, I've bought you several; that's something I like, choosing sexy lingerie.

I love to chat with the saleslady, describing the woman for whom the gift is intended; the mixture of legitimate discussion and sexual subtext fosters a kind of complicity that can quickly lead to the question: And if it were for you, which would you choose?

I might ask you to caress one of your breasts, lightly to brush the nipple with your fingertips through the dress and bra, as discreetly as possible. Another thing I love, that we both love to do together: to look at women and imagine their nipples. Their pussies, too, as it happens, but let's not get carried away: for the moment we're dealing with nipples. As I have several times had occasion to explain to lingerie saleswomen, so that they might better advise me, yours are rather special; they look as if they had been put together inside out, with the tip pointing inward, and they pop up, like little animals from their lairs, when aroused. I suppose that's what they're doing right now; you don't even need to touch them. Don't touch them. Interrupt the gesture you had perhaps begun, leave your hand suspended in the air, and content yourself with *thinking* about your breasts. Visualize them. As I've already explained, it's an extremely effective yoga technique (although its effectiveness is ordinarily put to other uses): visualizing a part of the body with the utmost precision, then projecting yourself there in thought and sensation. Weight, warmth, the different textures of the areolae and the surrounding skin, the border between the skin and the areolae … you are completely present in your breasts. As you read this, someone sitting across from you – but is someone sitting across from you? – should see the tips jutting up beneath the layers of cloth, as if you were wearing a wet T-shirt.

Again, stop. Put the newspaper aside. Think only about your breasts, and about me thinking about them, for fifteen minutes. You may close your eyes or not, as you please.

Was it good?

You thought about my hands on your breasts? That's what I thought about. Actually, my hands not *on* your breasts, but *near* them. You know: the palms cupping and following their curve; a fraction of an inch closer and they would graze your breasts but that's just it, they don't. 'Graze' means 'to touch lightly'. Well, I'm not touching you, I'm getting as close as possible without making contact. The game consists precisely of keeping my distance, a constant distance requiring infinitesimal retractions of the palm in response to the breast as it moves, affected by arousal or simply by your breathing. When I say 'in response', it's more subtle than that, it's not a question of responding, which would be too late. As in the martial arts, where the object is not to parry a blow but to avoid receiving it, one must learn to anticipate, letting oneself be guided by intuition, bodily warmth, breath, with practice reaching a point where the tip of the breast and the hollow of the palm operate like two galvanic fields. And you and I have had considerable practice. Touché, you lose. This can be done with any part of the body, moreover, and although palms and fingers, lips and tongues, breasts, clitoris, glans and anus are clearly the time-tested combinations, the ones that within minutes provoke cries that can drive neighbours insane (trying not to cry out isn't bad either), it would be a mistake to stick to the classic erogenous zones, neglecting variations like the scalp/hollow-behind-the-knee combo, chin/sole of the foot, hip bone/armpit (I am a devotee of the armpit and in particular of yours, which is just on the tip of my tongue, so to speak).

That makes you smile because you know how I adore armpits, whereas you, you've got nothing against them but it's not what turns you inside out. My enthusiasm warms your heart more than it heats you up. So: you are smiling. Writing this, two months before you read it – assuming all goes as planned – I try to imagine that smile, the smile of a woman on a train, reading a graphic porno letter addressed to her yet read at the same time by thousands of other women and thinking to herself, I suppose, that she's really lucky. It's an unusual situation, admittedly, which no doubt provokes an unusual smile, and I find that evoking such a smile is an exhilarating literary ambition. I like literature to be effective; ideally, I want it to be performative, in the sense in which linguists define a performative statement, the classic example being the sentence 'I declare war', which instantly means war has been declared. One might argue that of all literary genres, pornography is the one that most closely approaches that ideal: reading 'You're getting wet', makes you get wet.

That was only an example: I did not say 'You're getting wet', so you should not be getting wet now, and if you are, pay no attention to it, concentrate on something other than your panties. There's a story I like, it's about this guy, and a magician promises to grant all his wishes, on one condition: for five minutes he must not think about a pink elephant. Which he would never have thought about, of course, but once it's been mentioned and forbidden, how can he think of anything else? Still, I'll try to help you; we'll think of something else, we'll turn our attention to your armpits. We'll even *do* something else.

You are now entitled to a little contact. While continuing to hold the paper in your left hand, you will place your right hand on your left hip. Your forearm, which I assume is bare, should be resting on your belly, over your navel. Move your hand up from the hip to the little bulge all women have directly above the waistband of their skirt or trousers and gently rub the warm, tender and elastic flesh there. A soft, relaxing sensation; a base camp where it would be nice to linger. So linger a moment before continuing the ascent towards the ribs and the bottom of your bra. At this stage, the situation might vary a little, depending on whether a second layer of clothing – blouse over T-shirt, light jacket – allows you to operate relatively clandestinely or requires you to advance in the open. In any case, you can always position the hand holding the paper to screen the one now frankly cradling your left breast. There, you have free rein. Take as long as you want and do – within the bounds of decency – everything you wanted to do earlier, when contact was forbidden. But don't forget that our current objective is not the nipple, but the armpit towards which your fingers are pointing. There you will surely have access to your bare skin via the armhole of the dress or T-shirt, and if you happen to be wearing a long-sleeved blouse, you'll have to go in through the neckline, which I assume is low-cut. Whatever route you take, from above or below, for the first time since you began reading, you are now touching your skin. Move your left arm a little away from your body; it will look quite natural if you lean your elbow on the armrest. With your fingertips, stroke your shoulder, then begin to explore the hollow of your armpit. On a July afternoon, in what I imagine is a rather crowded train, I'd be surprised if you don't find a few drops of sweat. I would like you, in a few minutes – above all, don't hurry – to bring them to your nose, to smell, then to your lips, to taste. I adore that. Without going to extremes, I'm not crazy about well-scrubbed skin, and you're the same way, you like the smells of sex: dick, pussy, armpit. Your underarms aren't shaved, I love that too. Not as a general rule, it's not a requirement, more of a case-by-case thing, but in your case, absolutely. I could spend hours – in fact I do spend hours – in that light pelt of blonde fur. This belongs, as you've pointed out, to an ensemble of erotic preferences that places me more in the chic-sleazy mode of Jean-François Jonvelle's photos, let's say, than in the harder line of Helmut Newton's. The girl in skimpy panties who massages her breasts with moisturizing lotion while smiling at you in the bathroom mirror, rather than the ambiance of spike heels, dog collar and disdainful pout. But there's more than that in the taste for underarm hair; there is also – how to put it? – a kind of metonymical effect, as when one says 'crown' to mean 'monarchy', the idea that you walk around with two little extra pussies, two little pussies you're allowed to display in public even though they're irresistibly reminiscent, for me anyway, of the one between your legs. In theory, I disapprove of this sort of thing. Presented with a pussy, I'm for thinking about that pussy, and with an armpit, that armpit. Postulating that everything corresponds to everything else in a system of ineffable echoes and correlations –

that can lead to romanticism, from romanticism to bovarysm, and from there to the generalized denial of the real. I am for the real, nothing but the real, and for taking care of one thing at a time, like the Indian guru who, in another of my favourite stories, tirelessly repeats to his disciples: 'When you eat, eat. When you read, read. When you walk, walk. When you make love, make love,' and so on. Except that one day, during a meditation session, his disciples find him eating his breakfast while reading the newspaper. When they are astonished, the guru replies, 'What's the problem? When you eat and read, eat and read.' I cite that example when, counter to my philosophical beliefs, I think of your pussy while caressing and having you caress your armpits, and what's more you're thinking of it too and I won't mention that passenger over there who's been watching you for five minutes out of the corner of his eye as you lick your fingers.

For the moment, no, I won't mention him.

Another inexhaustible marvel: not only are women naked under their clothes, but they all have that miraculous thing between their legs, and the most unsettling part is that they have it all the time, even without thinking about it. For a long while, I wondered how they managed; in their place, I felt, I'd be masturbating non-stop, or at least considering it. One of the things about you that pleased me right away is the impression that you think about it more than the average woman. Somebody once told you that you wore your pussy on your face; you hesitated over how to take that, as a compliment, or leering vulgarity, and opted in the end for the compliment. I agree. I like it that looking at a woman's face, one can imagine her coming. Some women, it's just about impossible, there's no hint of abandonment, but you, watching you move, smile, talk about something entirely unrelated, one guesses right away that you love to come. One wants immediately to know what you're like when you do and I'm here to say that, well, one is not disappointed. Although it isn't really in the tone of this piece, I'll allow myself a sentimental aside: I have never enjoyed so much seeing someone come, and when I say 'seeing', of course, it isn't just seeing. I imagine you reading this: your smile, your pride, the pride of a well-laid woman, equalled only by that of the man who lays a well-laid woman. You can shove your thoughts into your panties now. But wait, don't be in a rush. Try the pink elephant trick. Don't think yet about my dick, or my tongue, or my fingers, or yours; think about your pussy all alone, the way it is now between your legs. It's truly difficult, what I'm asking of you here, but the idea is to think of your pussy as if you were not thinking of it. People who meditate a lot say that the goal – and illumination is strictly a bonus – is to observe one's breathing without changing it in any way. To be there as if one were not there. Try to imagine your pussy from the inside, as if it were simply between your legs and you were thinking about something else, as if you were busy working or reading an article on the new members of the European Community. Try to remain neutral, indifferent, yet consider every sensation. The way the fabric of your panties compresses your bush. The labia majora. The labia minora. The contact of the folds, one against another. Close your eyes.

Ah? You're wet? I rather suspected that. Very wet? I admit that the exercise was difficult, but, well, wet though you may be, your pussy isn't open. You're sitting on a train, wearing panties, and haven't yet slipped in a finger, so it can't be open. Listen, now we'll see if it's possible to spread those interior labia a little bit, all by themselves. I don't know. I don't think so. You have excellent vaginal muscles but they don't control the opening of the labia; what you can do, on the other hand, is grip and relax, grip and relax, as hard as you can, as if I were inside you.

There, I skipped ahead a bit, I went faster than I intended, but it would be unkind to rewind. You therefore have the right to think about my dick. But without pouncing on it. Take your time. I'm sure all you can think about is thrusting it inside you up to the hilt and masturbating at the same time, but you'll have to be patient, to follow my rhythm, which is basically always to slow down, delay, hold back. I was a premature ejaculator in my youth; it's an awful experience that convinced me that the greatest pleasure is to be always on the verge of pleasure. That's where I love to be, precisely *on the verge*, and I love to keep pushing back that edge, always sharpening the point a little more. At first you found that a bit disturbing; now, no. Now you love it when, before licking you, I caress your clitoris for a long time with just the warmth of my breath, by breathing close by, drawing out the wait for the first lick. You love it when, before going in full length, I stay for a long time with the head right at the entrance. You love to tell me, looking straight into my eyes, that you love my dick in your pussy; you love to say it over and over and that's what you'll do now. There, on the train. You'll say: I want your dick in my pussy – in a very low voice, obviously, but say it, don't just think it, form the sounds with your lips. Pronounce these words as *loudly* as you can without the other passengers hearing you. Seek the sound threshold and draw as close as you can without crossing it. You've seen someone saying the rosary. Do the same thing, the basic mantra being 'I want your dick in my pussy'. All variations are welcome and I expect you to give carte blanche to your imagination. Go to it. Until Poitiers, which shouldn't be too far now, if my calculations are correct.

Meanwhile, I'm thinking about your fellow passengers. True, I'm of two minds about these people, whom I'm tempted to put to use but who are dangerously outside my control. I'm aware, also, that this letter seems like both a delightful object of pure pleasure and the disturbing device of a confirmed control freak. If everything has gone as planned, you are reading this page on Saturday, 20 July, at around 4.15, the train having just left the station after its stop in Poitiers. In fact, I wrote this page at the end of May, before leaving to shoot my film in Russia. When I asked the people at *Le Monde* early on to fix the publication date, they didn't understand why it was so important to me, so I told them what I told you: that it was a story of anticipation and that to anticipate I needed a precise target. That was true. I knew I'd be with my sons on the Île de Ré in mid-July and that you would arrive there a week later. The special section appears on Saturdays, and I knew you would have to take the train today, on this particular Saturday – but not before two o'clock, when *Le Monde* would definitely be at news-stands. I was careful to reserve your ticket in advance, hoping it would be difficult to change it during the holiday period. So we can say that, like the OCD veteran I am, I stacked the deck in my favour. Which doesn't prevent me from knowing, like every good obsessive, that I'm playing against chance, the unexpected, everything that can foul up the best of plans. An unbearable thought.

Writing this brought me immense pleasure, but also agonies of worry – which doubtless heightened the pleasure. I saw time stretching from point A to point B: at A, I send the piece in to *Le Monde*, it's out of my hands, I can't turn back, the die is cast – while B is the end of the line, you've finished reading, I'm waiting for you on the station platform, you are wild with desire and gratitude, everything has gone exactly as I'd dreamed. Between A, the end of May, and B, 5.45 on 20 July 2002, anything can happen, and trust me, I've imagined everything, from hapless screw-ups to hopeless catastrophes. That the trains would go on strike, or the newspapers. That you'd miss the train or it would jump the tracks. That you would no longer love me, or I you, that we'd no longer be together and my light-hearted scheme would become something sad or, even worse, embarrassing.

Only a man immune to superstition could plan his pleasure in such detail without fear of defying the gods. Imagine: you're a god, and a mortal comes along to tell you: Here's the thing, today, Thursday, 23 May, I've decided that on Saturday, 20 July, on the 2.45 train to La Rochelle, the woman I am in love with will masturbate according to my instructions and reach orgasm between Niort and Surgères – now how would you take that? I think you'd think: Well, he's got some nerve. Cute, but some nerve. You'd say to yourself that a little lesson was in order. Not the lightning bolt that zaps the reckless fool, nor the liver-devouring vulture, but still, a lesson. What kind of lesson? Myself, I believe that in your place – you're a god, remember – I'd try to arrange something along the lines of a Lubitsch film, where the audience always gets what it wants, but never in the way it wanted. And to give this overworked set-up the unexpected twist that both foils and fulfils expectations, Lubitsch would call on one of your fellow passengers. Who might be, for example, deaf. Can you imagine, a pretty, young deaf woman who for ten minutes has been slyly watching the lips of the woman next to her on the train as she whispers ecstatically, her eyes closed: 'I want your dick in my pussy'? To develop the scene, there's a wide range of possibilities, from a light, graceful moment of girlish confusion to the most extravagant sexual encounter. Now, if the idea is to teach me a lesson by nudging your sexual pleasure beyond my control and diverting it towards an unexpected beneficiary, the pretty deaf girl should morph into a pretty deaf *boy* – but that, as you can again imagine, thrills me considerably less. Let's move on, especially since I've thought of another possible scenario.

In real life, a writer might sometimes see a stranger reading his book in a public place, but that doesn't happen often; it's not something you can count on. Quite a few passengers on this train certainly do read *Le Monde*, however. Let's do the maths. France has 60 million inhabitants; *Le Monde*'s print run is 600,000 copies; its readers thus represent 1 per cent of the population. The proportion of readers on the Paris–La Rochelle high-speed train on a Saturday afternoon in July must be much higher, and I'd be tempted to jump it up to 10 per cent. So we get roughly 10 per cent of the passengers, most of whom – because today they have the time – will at least take a look at the short-story supplement, just to see. I don't want to seem immodest, but the chances of these just-taking-a-look passengers reading all the way to the end hover in my opinion around 100 per cent, for the simple reason that when there's ass involved, people read to the end; that's how it is. So about 10 per cent of your fellow passengers are reading, have read, or will read these instructions during the three hours you will all spend on the train. That's a completely different order of probability to that of having a pretty deaf woman sitting next to you. There's a one-in-ten chance – I'm probably exaggerating but not by much – that the person beside you is at this moment reading the same thing you are. And if not the person next to you, someone close by.

Don't you think the moment has come to go to the bar car? Roll up the section, tuck it into your handbag, rise, and start making your way through the train. I'll wait for you in the bar car. Don't take the story out again until you get there.

So. You stood in line, ordered a coffee or mineral water. There's a crowd in the bar car. You've managed to find a place on a stool, though, and spread the section out in front of you on the grey plastic counter; now you're reading again. While you were moving through the cars, did the same idea I had occur to you? Someone else on this train is reading this story. He reads, perhaps he smiles while reading, perhaps he thinks: Hey, this is a hoot, what's got into those guys at *Le Monde*? And then he does a doubletake on the 2.45 Paris–La Rochelle high-speed train on Saturday, 20 July. Eyebrows raised, he looks up from his paper, has a little moment of … vertigo would be too strong, but confusion, let's say. He rereads the sentence and thinks: Wait a minute, that's my train! And a moment later: Then the girl, the one he wrote this for, she's here too, on this train! Put yourself in this passenger's place, man or woman. Wouldn't you find that exciting? Wouldn't you try to find her, this girl? You have very little physical description, I was careful about that, but you do have a clue, and quite a precise one: you know that between Poitiers and Niort, i.e. between 4.15 and 4.45, she should be in the bar car. So what do you do? You go there. Me, anyway, I'd go. Ladies, gentlemen, be my guests. Don't sit around twiddling your thumbs: take your copy of *Le Monde* to show you're playing along and head for the bar.

I don't know if you've shown up here fully aware of the implications or whether you're realizing them only now, and I don't know what you think about this whole situation personally, but I love it.

What I like is that unlike the scene with the pretty, deaf woman, it has nothing to do with chance but proceeds automatically from the mechanism already set in motion. If the story has been published on the appointed day, if the train is indeed running that day, if the bar car is not closed, then it's certain – or I give up – that a few of the men and, I hope, women on the train will turn up on time, meaning *now*, hoping to identify you. They are there, around you. I don't know them, but I summoned them two months ago and here they are. How's that for performative literature?!

Even though you are something of an exhibitionist, I imagine that you have now buried your nose in the paper and don't dare look up. Look up a little. You are facing the window. If it were night-time, or if the train were streaking through a tunnel, the car interior would be reflected in the window and you could see *them* without turning round, but there is no tunnel, no reflection, only the dreary landscape of the Vendée: water towers, low houses, towpaths beneath a sun still high in the sky.

And *them*, behind you.

Come on. No use keeping your head in the sand.

Take a deep breath, then turn round.

Innocently, casually.

Go on.

They are all here.

Men, women. Trying to look innocent, like you, but several are holding *Le Monde*.

Are they looking at you?

I'm sure they're looking at you. I'm sure they've been looking at you for several minutes; didn't you feel their eyes on your back? They were waiting for you to turn round, and now, you're facing them, it's as if you were naked in front of them.

Do you think this has gone too far? That things are beginning to resemble a scene in a horror movie? The heroine believes she has taken refuge in a safe place, a crowded bar car, when a seemingly harmless detail suddenly reveals that the people around her, also seemingly harmless, are all part of the conspiracy. Spies, zombies, alien invaders, it doesn't matter – they all read *Le Monde*, that's what identifies them, and now they surround her, closing in …

Do you feel caught in a trap?

Just joking. That's not where this story is going. Think about it. First off, you are not the only suspect: I'm sure that other women in the bar are carrying prominently displayed copies of *Le Monde*. How many? One, four, eleven? Three or more I'll consider a real success. Not only did I ask these women to come here – as many of them as possible and preferably alone, so as not to cede the terrain to a horde of men – I also asked for something else. Well, I'm asking them now, actually, but I strongly suspect that, unlike you, they have not strictly followed the story's instructions, so they have reached this paragraph ahead of you. This is what I ask of them: if you have read this letter and found it arousing, even just a little, then play the game; during the last hour of the trip, between Niort and La Rochelle, behave as if you were the intended recipient. The role is simple: read *Le Monde* while drinking coffee or mineral water in the bar car and pay attention to what is happening around you. Simple, yes, but it can be extremely sexy. I'm counting on your help.

There, everything is ready. I'll go over the rules again. In the bar car, a certain number of men and women have read this story and are, with various motives, all essentially sexual, trying to identify the heroine. That heroine is you, but only you know this, and the other women are pretending to be you. The heroine has been achingly wet now for two hours, and the other women are following suit, but, unlike the heroine, they have read the whole story and therefore know what happens next.

I do love this situation. I love it that, thanks to *Le Monde*, it really exists, but I no longer see how to control it. Too many characters, too many variables. So I'm no longer in charge. I throw up my hands. I continue to imagine things, of course: a ballet of glances, discreet smiles, a wink among 'us girls'; a stifled giggle, perhaps a peal of laughter, possibly some extreme acting out or maybe a scandal, why not? Someone who says loud and clear that this is disgusting – and that he doesn't buy Hubert Beuve-Méry's paper to read such garbage; perhaps a sharp, sophisticated exchange along the lines of I-know-that-you-know-that-I-know, or maybe two strangers who come to the bar and then leave together. I wonder what the passengers who haven't read *Le Monde* are noticing. Anything? Do they sense that something is going on without knowing what? I wonder, I imagine, but I no longer decide: now I let everyone improvise his or her individual role, and I'm awaiting your arrival in an hour so you can tell me all about it in bed and later over a big platter of seafood, or maybe the other way round. You see, I'm not that bossy.

There are forty-five minutes left to the trip, and about a thousand words left for my story. Eight thousand is my limit. The other women readers of *Le Monde* already know what can still happen, outside of everything beyond my control, and you, naturally, have your suspicions. You saw one woman get up a few minutes ago, watched her leave, and noticed others were watching her, too. They all know what it means and she knows they know. It means: I am going to go get myself off.

So the woman leaves the bar car, heading for the closest toilet. Occupied. She waits a minute. Thinking she hears the sound of panting despite the racket of the train, she glues her ear to the door, and smiles. A man standing nearby in the corridor looks at her in some surprise; he's holding a different newspaper, and she thinks: Poor guy, he has no idea what he's missing. Finally the toilet door opens; a woman emerges with *Le Monde* sticking out of her bag. The two women exchange a look; the one leaving the toilet has come hard, the woman waiting sees it in her face and that excites her, so much that she asks boldly: Was it good? The first replies, very convincingly: Yes, it was, leaving the guy who doesn't have *Le Monde*, poor fellow, to think that something really screwy is going on in this train. The waiting woman goes in, locks the door. She looks at herself in the large mirror on the wall behind the sink, which allows her, when she lifts up her dress – or pulls down her trousers – to get a good view of what she is about to do. She takes off her wet panties, raises one leg and places a foot on the edge of the sink; with one hand she holds on to the grab bar, and begins touching her pussy with the other. She goes for it, fingers in, too late for dainty refinements, she wants it too much and has been ready for at least an hour now. She uses two fingers right away, shoves them in, it's dripping wet and gets wetter as she watches her hand go at her pussy in the mirror, fingers working away. Or perhaps she goes about it differently, starts with her clitoris: each woman has her own technique. I love that she's showing hers to me, and here I'm projecting yours on her; that doesn't matter. Maybe this is the first time she has masturbated standing in a train toilet, and it's certainly the first time she's done it knowing that people outside the door know what she's doing. It's as if she were doing it in front of everyone; she looks at her pussy in the mirror as if everybody were looking at it, as if they were watching her fingers sliding between her wet labia; it's incredibly exciting. She thinks about you, whom she hasn't identified for certain. Still, she has someone in mind: the tall blonde with the long neck, slender waist and ample hips, the one mentioned early in the story. Perhaps that was to put people off the scent, but maybe not, and there was one girl who really looked the part. The woman thinks that, given what time it is, you are probably in a toilet yourself, in another car, doing the same thing; she imagines your fingers thrusting through your blonde bush and even though she's not particularly interested in girls, at this point she'd go for that, really enjoy it. She's seeing her own fingers in her pussy, and yours in yours, and the fingers of other women in their pussies, all getting themselves off at the same time on the same train, all dripping wet, all closing in now on their clitorises – all because some guy, two months earlier, decided to take advantage of a commission from *Le Monde* to whip himself up a little erotic scenario with his girlfriend. Now she's there, her fingers are on her clitoris, she spreads the labia to get at it, to see it better in the mirror over the sink, and let's say she does it the way you do at this point, fingertips, index and middle fingers, rubbing harder and harder; she'd love to caress a nipple with the other hand, but she has to keep hold of the bar to steady herself. She looks at her face – it's rare to see oneself about to come – she wants to cry out, it's building fast, she knows there is someone outside the door, she knows she's breathing hard, making noise while someone's listening, but she's so close now, she wants to shout, she wants to say yes, she wants to shout yes! – she holds back from shouting yes when she comes but you hear her anyway, you are outside the door, you say yes too, yes, the train's pulling into Surgères; now, at last, it's your turn.

Back in your seat, just before the train pulls into La Rochelle, you read the last paragraph, in which I invite all the men and women who made the trip, on the train or elsewhere, to tell me about their experiences. Perhaps that will lead to a sequel, which will be not only performative but interactive. What could be better than that? I even give them my e-mail address: emmanuelcarrere@yahoo.fr. You think I've got some nerve. You're right, I've got some nerve. I'm waiting for you on the platform. ■

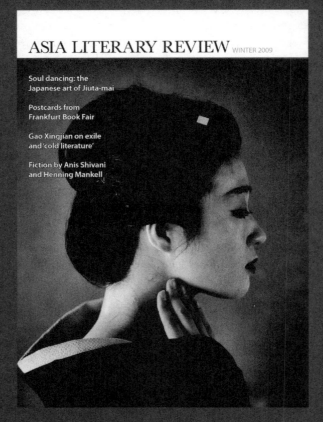

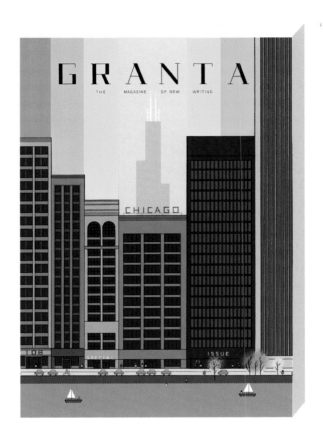

BODY

Yann Faucher

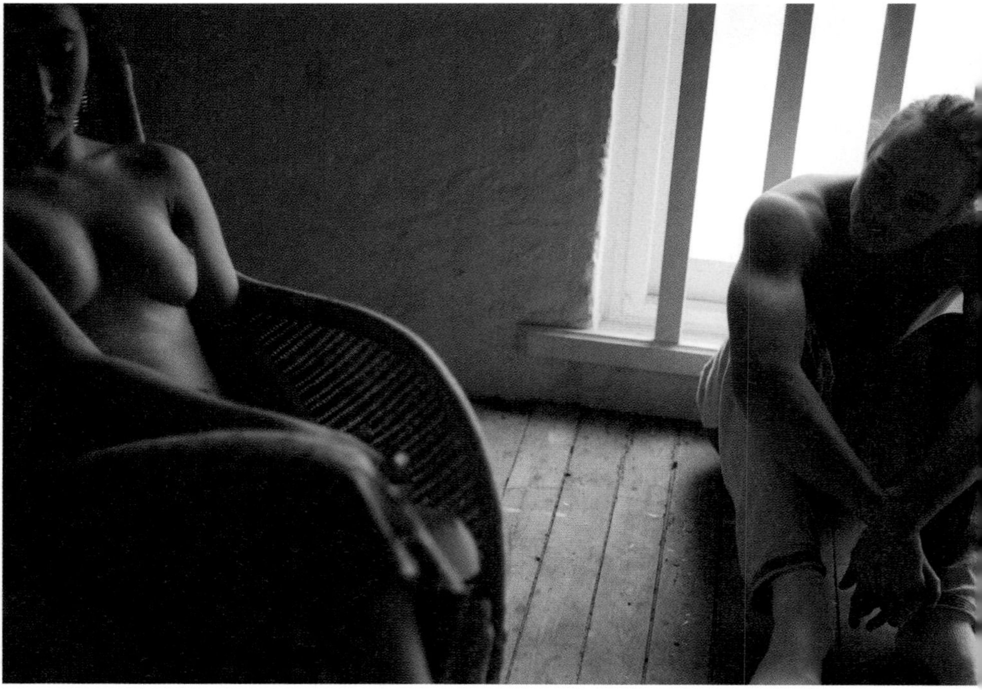

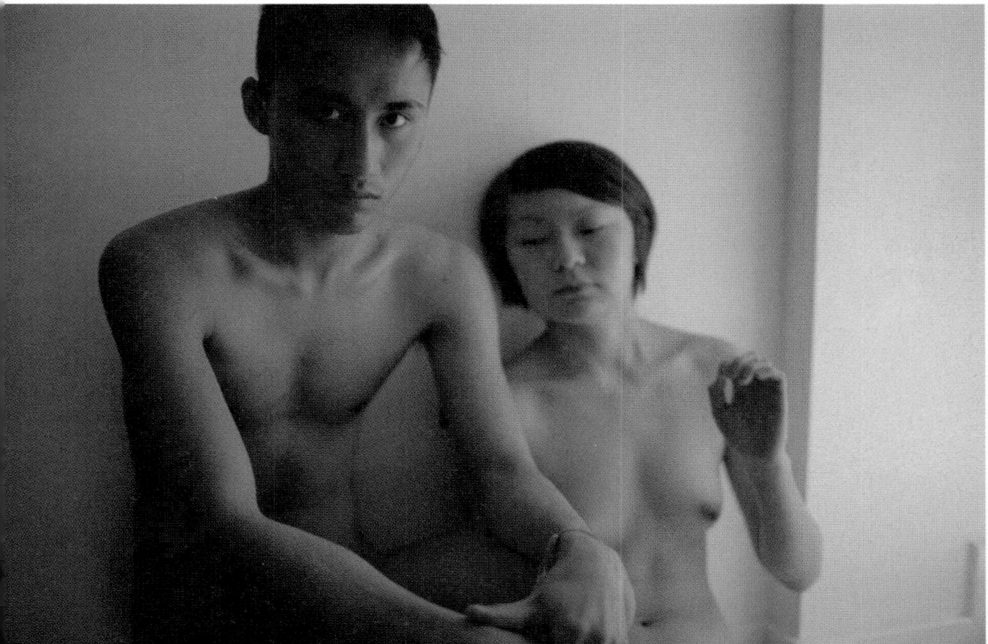

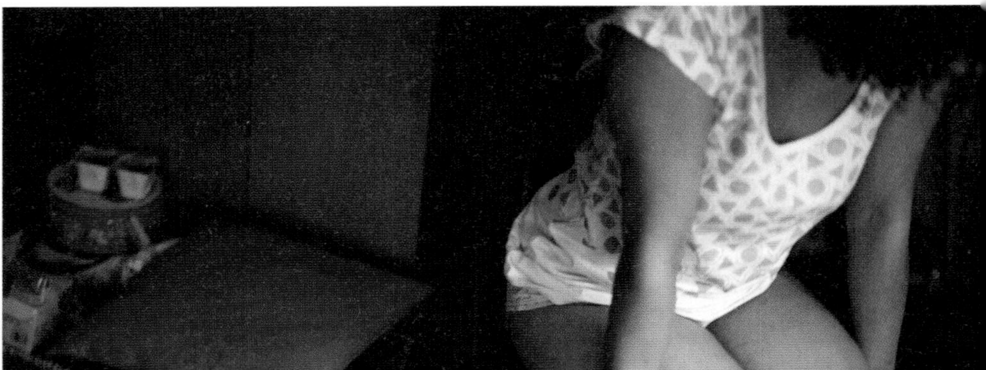
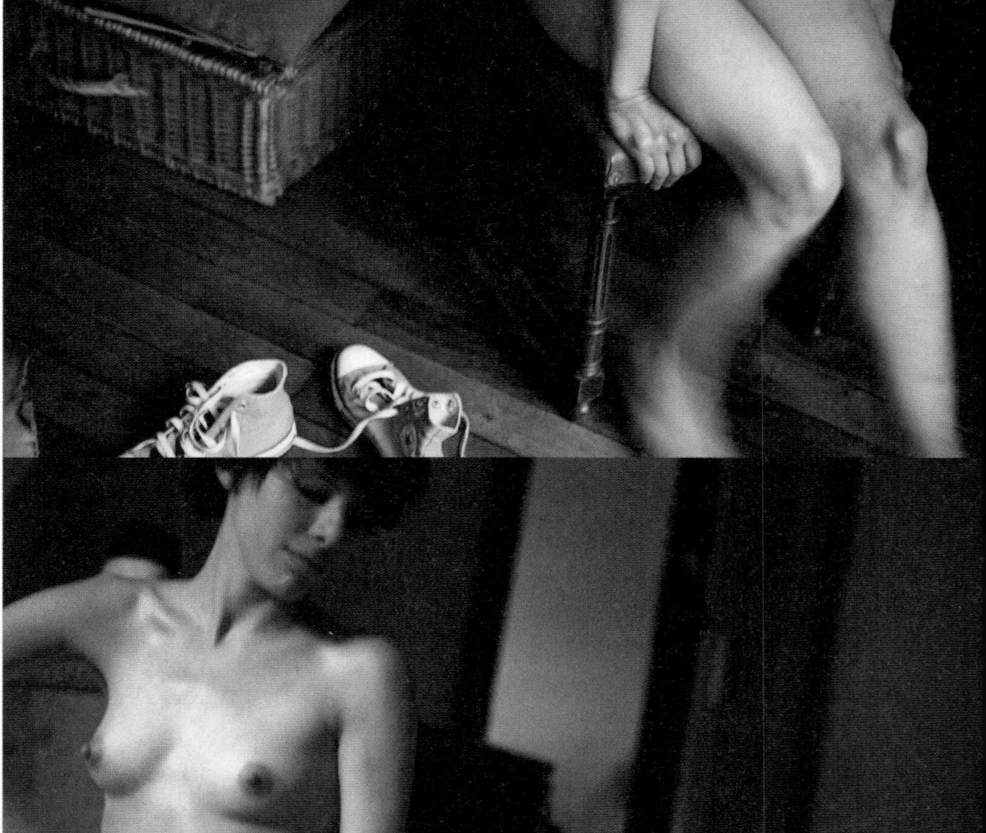

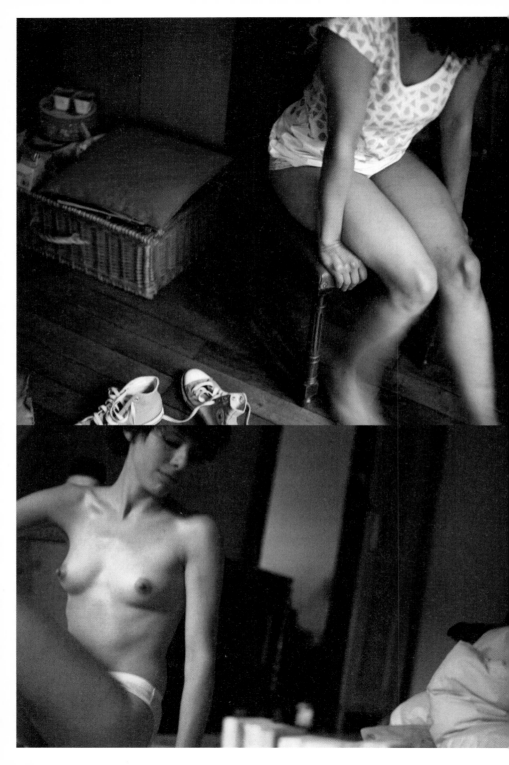

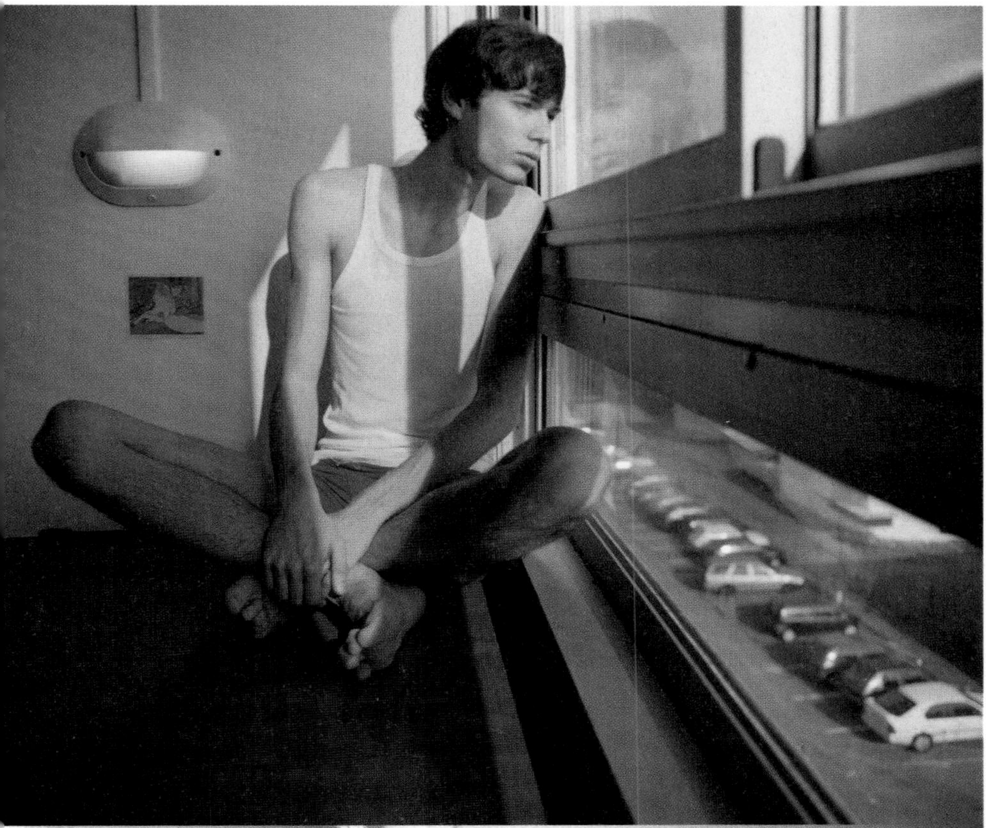

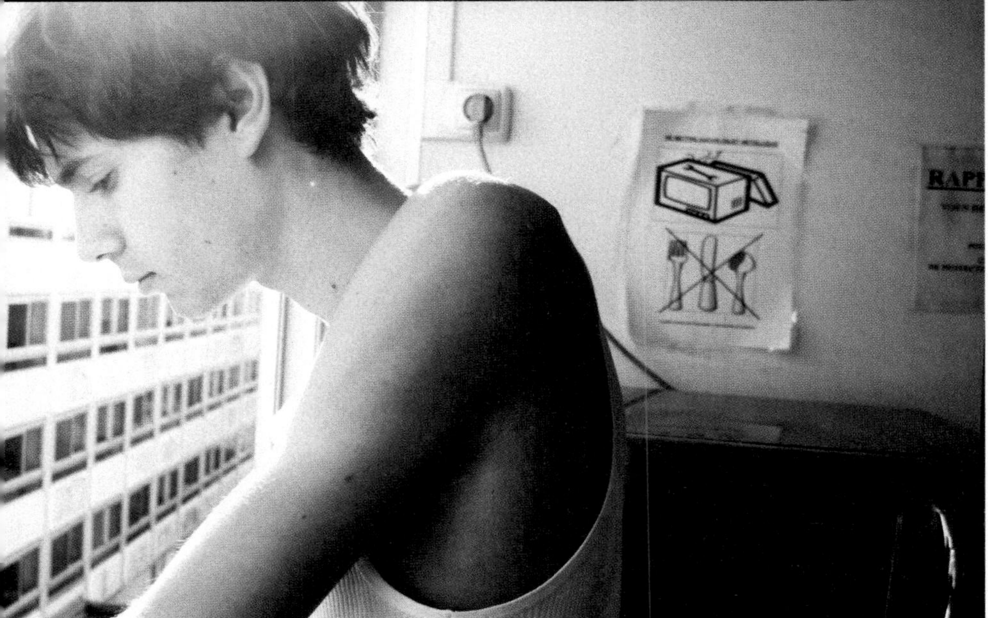

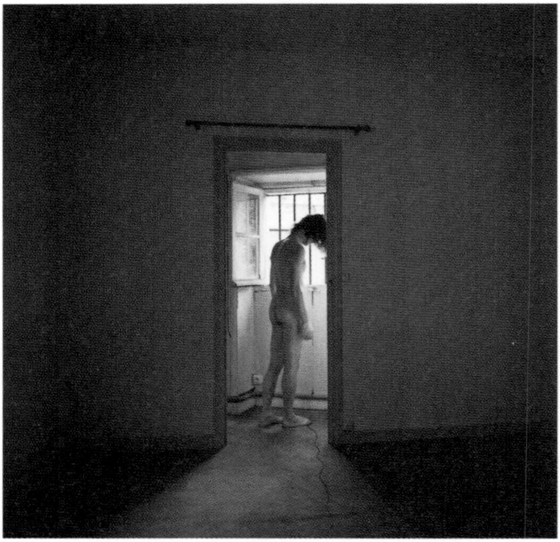

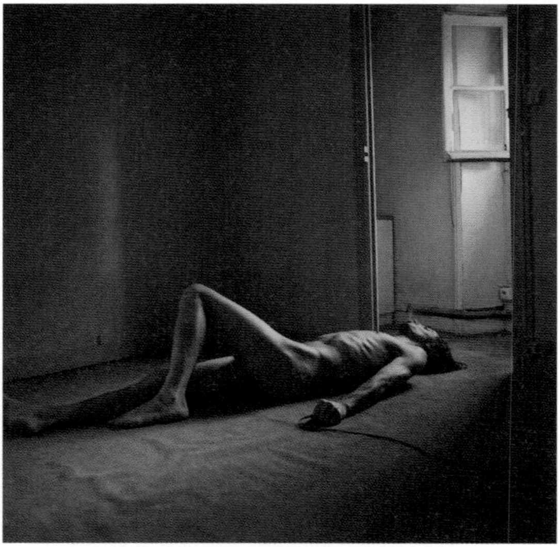

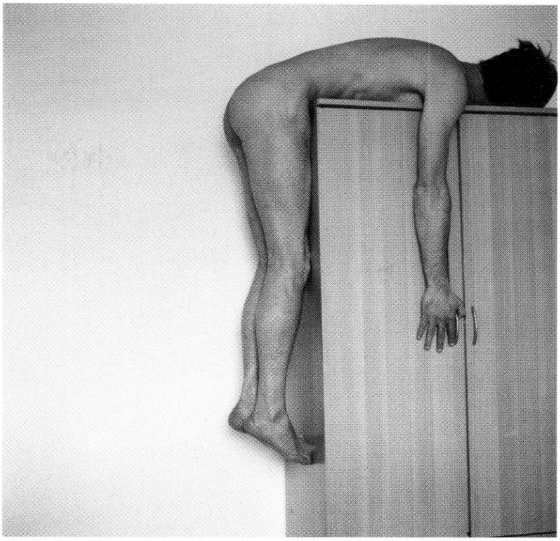

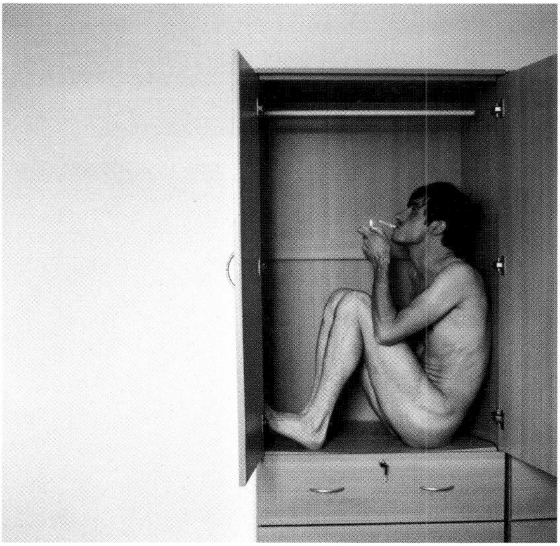

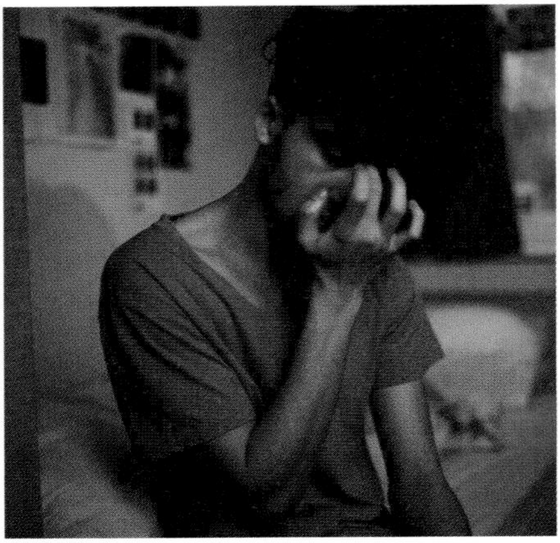
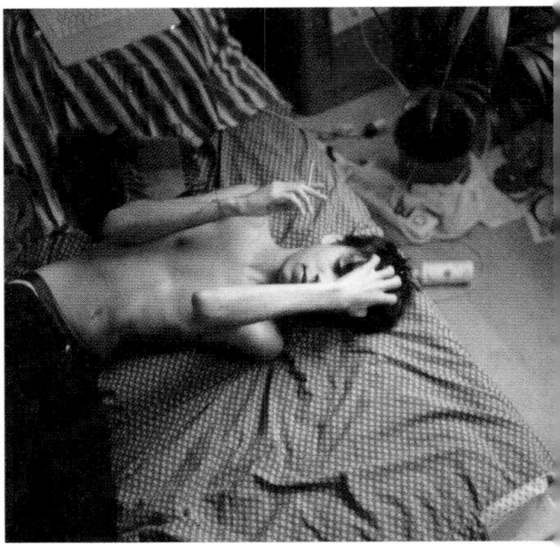
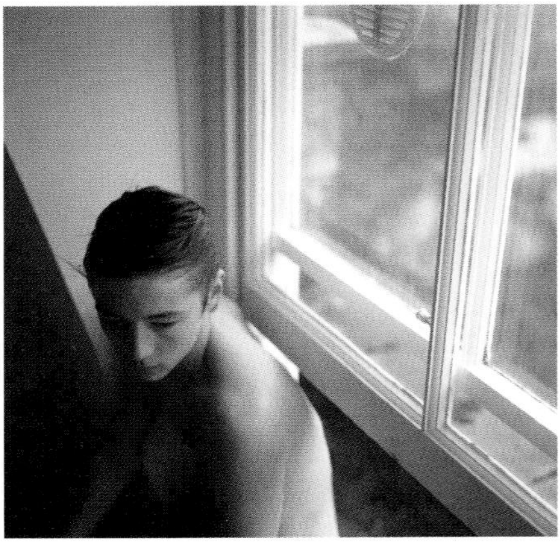
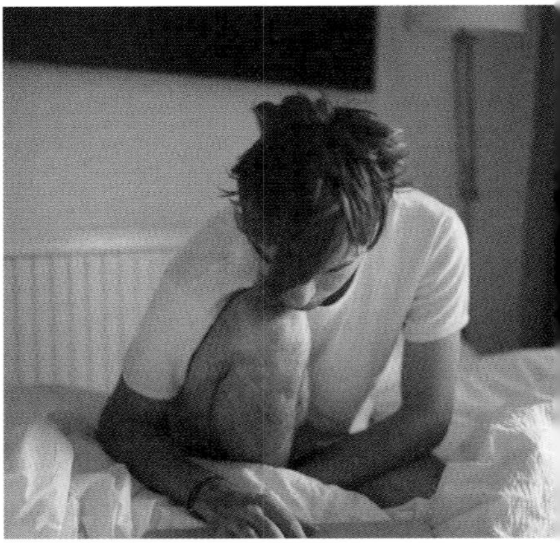
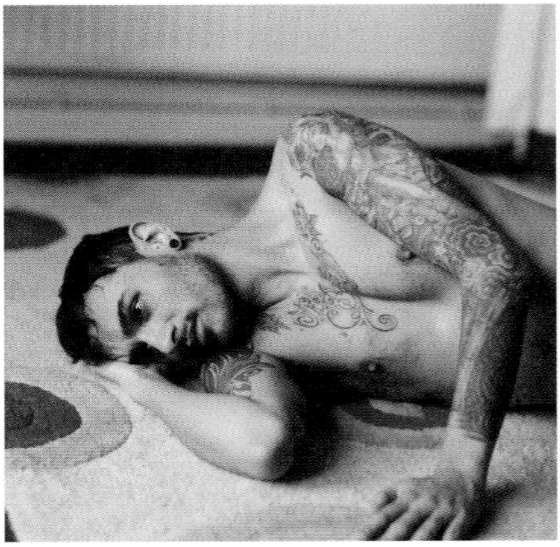
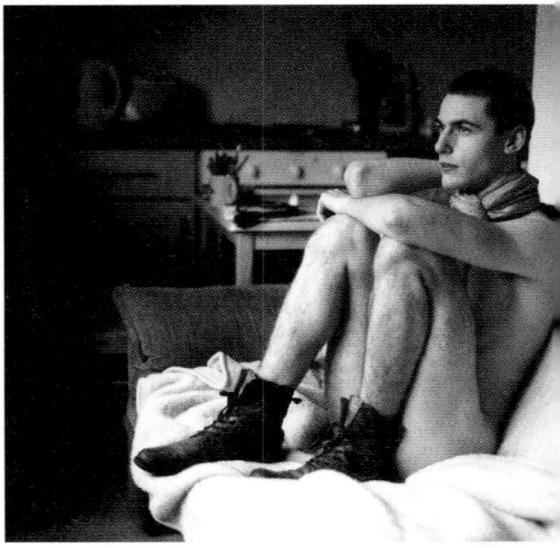

PARK LIFE

Rupert Thomson

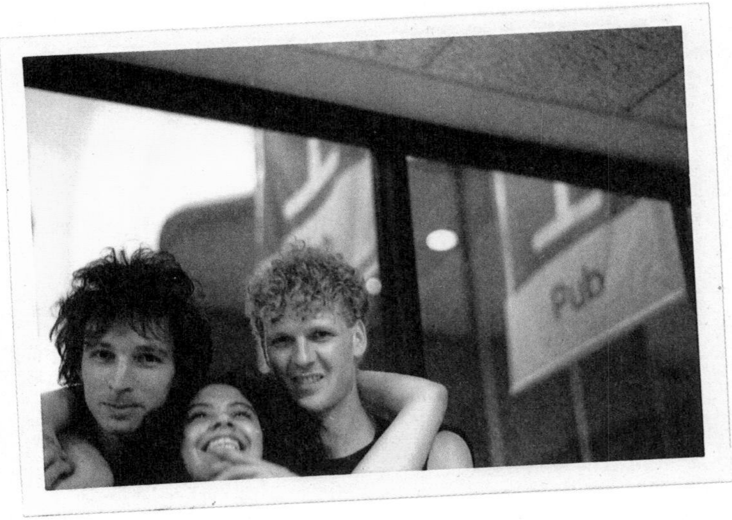
Pub

I flew into JFK at the end of December 1984, and as soon as I saw the giant floodlit billboards stacking up in front of the Triborough Bridge the blood began to hiss and crackle in my veins. At that time, New York was my favourite place: it was everything a city should be – a volatile mix of edginess and possibility.

My father had died a few months before and I had inherited some money, but it wasn't enough to live on. I knew I would have to find work quickly. At a New Year's Eve party on the Upper West Side, a pretty blonde girl told me I should apply to a bookstore called the Strand. 'They take all kinds of people,' she said. I wasn't sure whether or not this was a compliment – it didn't sound like one – but I followed her advice, and within a few days I had a job. The pay was $125 a week.

Like most Strand employees, I started in the Review Books section, which was in the basement. Though winter gripped the city, it was hot and dusty down there, and I spent my first days sorting and shelving hardback editions of novels that had just been published. *All kinds of people*, the blonde girl had said, and now I understood what she meant: never in my life had I come across such an extravagant array of misfits, bohemians and would-be artists, which more than made up for the dismal salary and the dullness of the job. There was a thin-wristed, moon-pale DJ from Arkansas who spoke in a sardonic voice that made me think of Flannery O'Connor. There was a timid, bespectacled man who ate cake secretly in the downstairs toilet. There was a sweet-natured older man with shoulder-length grey hair, who smoked with great purpose despite his chronic emphysema. There was a winsome, bruised-looking transsexual by the name of Opal. And then there was Klaus, from Vienna. An ex-junkie and sometime lead guitarist, Klaus was the only other 'European' in the store. He was working illegally as I was – we were both using Social Security numbers that we had borrowed from close friends – and it wasn't long before we were meeting for drinks, usually in the Holiday

Lounge, a dive bar in the East Village. Later, we would go back to Klaus's apartment, which was on 51st Street, between Seventh and Broadway, and which he shared with a six-foot-tall, black-eyed Venezuelan girl who stayed up all night doing coke. Klaus and I soon became so inseparable that people in-store started calling us 'The Two Musketeers'.

It was everyone's ambition to get out of Review Books, and when Klaus asked if I would be interested in the graveyard detail I jumped at the chance. Graveyard details worked like this. When people who owned books died in New York, a member of the family would often call the Strand and offer to sell the library as a job lot. The Strand would then send an assessor to the home of the deceased, and a price would be agreed. Some days later, two employees would be dispatched in the Strand van, and the books would be loaded into boxes and taken back to the store. The van was the same shade of red as the famous Strand T-shirt, and it was driven by Nelson, a former Hell's Angel with a plaited ponytail that hung heavily between his shoulder blades. Gears clashing, he would slam through the Manhattan traffic while Klaus and I bounced around in the back on bound stacks of cardboard flats. Nelson had a gruff manner and most people were afraid of him – even the boss treated him with a respect that seemed out of proportion to his job – but something about us 'Europeans' seemed to entertain him.

One particular graveyard detail sticks in my mind, perhaps because we happened to go to an address on West 80th Street, only yards from the building where I was staying. As Klaus and I climbed the stairs to the sixth floor, we were accompanied by one of the dead woman's relatives – a cousin, I think, or a nephew – and he explained that she had lived alone for many years, and that we shouldn't be too surprised by what we found. I didn't know it at the time, but the apartment I entered that afternoon was a classic example of syllogomania, or Diogenes syndrome, a condition common among the elderly who live on their own. They lose the ability to throw things away, and gradually the line between possessions and rubbish begins to blur. The narrow corridor that ran through the middle of the apartment was narrowed still further by the newspapers and plastic bags that had piled up on either side, almost to the ceiling. In the living room, several items of furniture had been buried completely; imprinted in the junk that had accumulated on the couch was the shape of the woman's body, like a hare's form. We had to guess where the bookshelves might be, and then burrow our way through to them. Later, the woman's relative asked if we wanted to take anything from the apartment in exchange for all our hard work. I chose a large, framed black-and-white photograph of a gala night at the Waldorf-Astoria that had been taken the year I was born.

In late March, and possibly on Nelson's say-so, Klaus and I were offered the job of running the Strand's kiosk in Bryant Park. We accepted at once. This was before Giuliani sanitized – or rather, ruined – Times Square, and though Bryant Park was bounded in the east by the austere edifice of the New York Public Library, the poky strip clubs and fizzing neon signs of 42nd Street weren't far away. From now on, we would be spending our days outdoors, in the vivid, grubby heart of the city.

Once we had punched in at the Strand at nine in the morning, we would load boxes of books into the back of the van – these were to replace the stock we had sold the day before – and then Nelson would drive us up to the park. The first hour was spent setting up – unlocking the kiosk, erecting the trestle tables, and laying out the books, spine uppermost. While one of us carried the tables out on to the paved area, the other would walk over to a diner on Sixth Avenue and bring back coffee and pumpernickel bagels with cream cheese. Most of the selling was accomplished between the hours of eleven and four, with peak activity occurring at lunchtime, when the office workers spilled out of high-rises like the Grace Building and strolled beneath the trees or perched on the smooth stone lip of the fountain. At the end of the day we would pack away the tables and the books, lock up the kiosk, and take the subway back to the store. If the weather was poor, we'd close early.

As the weeks went by, I began to realize that the park had its own unofficial and carefully calibrated infrastructure. The main business of the park was drugs, and the area was divided into four quadrants, each of which was patrolled by a different gang. Every gang had a captain. Usually black guys in their twenties or early thirties, they exuded an air of casual authority: this was their turf. Their underlings would loiter nearby, sometimes venturing out on to the sidewalk, sometimes hanging back, but always watching, circling. 'Sense, sense' was the perennial, muttered chant, sinsemilla being the drug of choice in Bryant Park, the female flowers of the cannabis plant glistening brownish-green inside their see-through plastic packets, like the crushed backs of cockroaches. But the dealers weren't the only regular fixtures in the park. At right angles to our kiosk, and backing on to Sixth Avenue, were two other kiosks run by three brothers from New Jersey. They were a little older than us, in their mid- to late thirties – Roy, Nick and Jake, and a beautiful Puerto Rican friend of theirs, Maritza, who would eventually, and disastrously, marry Klaus and move to Vienna with him. Like us, the brothers traded in second-hand books, but they had also branched out into postcards, calendars and maps. Though cagey at first, they quickly became good friends, and would invite us to yard parties in Hoboken, where there would be beer and joints and music, and where Roy would invariably perform his notorious snake dance. Stationed opposite our kiosk was a guy called Billy who sold hot dogs, soft drinks and bags of potato chips out of a metallic silver cart. He had thick blond hair, and wore check shirts and jeans. He smoked a lot of pot, and his eyes were often sleepy and bloodshot. He came from Brooklyn. Though amiable enough, he didn't exactly strike me as the sharpest tool in the box. Klaus thought Billy looked like an Austrian peasant, which was another way of saying the same thing.

In time we got to know most of the characters who passed through the park on a daily basis, but there was one who particularly intrigued us. He was in his forties, with a drooping moustache, and he wore aviator-style sunglasses with brown tinted lenses. He dressed in a denim jacket and jeans, both of which looked ever so slightly too new. A bulky key chain dangled from his brown leather belt. He reminded me of an extra from a bad seventies movie. He rarely bought anything, but he would look at our books most days, and his outfit meant that he never went unnoticed. We wondered who he was and what he was up to; we didn't trust him. When we mentioned him to the brothers from Hoboken, they laughed so hard they almost fell off their upturned beer crates. The guy was an undercover detective, they told us, and his remit was to bust the drug gangs that operated in the area. As Roy said, he would have been less visible if he'd come dressed as a cop. Sometimes he would tip off the police by murmuring into a hidden mike, but even before the sirens could be heard, the black guys would be scattering in all directions, like beads from a broken necklace, and by the time the cop cars surged over the sidewalk and rocked to a halt by the fountain, the gangs would be long gone. There would be a lot of posturing and shoulder-shrugging on the part of the police, and then, after buying a few cans of soda from Billy, they would drive away again.

I had already noticed that Billy didn't take any money from the dealers when he gave them soft drinks and potato chips, and I wondered if he was running some kind of tab, but then I happened to see one of the drug captains deftly drop a bag of sinsemilla into Billy's cart. While traders were making fortunes in stocks and shares on Wall Street, I was witness to a revival of the medieval barter system in Bryant Park. Up until that moment, we had been buying our grass from the Venezuelan girl who Klaus shared an apartment with, but now an idea occurred to me.

'Billy?' I said one steamy afternoon in May, while Klaus and I were sitting by the fountain. 'Do you like reading?'

'Yeah,' Billy said, 'I read.'

I asked if he would consider trading some of his grass for a few of our books.

He nodded slowly. 'That might work.'

'So have we got anything,' I said, 'that you might be interested in?'

He glanced towards our tables, and a kind of slow-motion shudder passed across his face as a thought surfaced in his brain.

'*The Collected Hegel*,' he said, 'in three volumes – I could go for that.'

I looked at Klaus, and we both burst out laughing.

'Is that a problem?' Billy said.

The three volumes, which were bound in green linen and tied with ribbon, were priced at something like $25, but the delicious way in which Billy had wrong-footed us meant that I didn't even give it a second thought.

'Billy,' I said, 'you've got a deal.'

This wasn't the first time we had worked an angle – but then, according to the brothers from Hoboken, all Strand employees worked an angle, especially if they were sent to Bryant Park. There was a story – possibly apocryphal – that the guy who had run the kiosk a year or two earlier had stolen so many books during the course of the summer that when he had left the Strand in the fall he had opened a bookstore of his own. Klaus and I were less flagrant. Most customers required a receipt when they purchased a book, but if they failed to ask for a receipt we would choose not to issue one, and the lack of evidence for that particular sale meant that we could pocket the cash and act as though the book in question had never existed. Since Klaus and I were responsible for choosing the stock that travelled up to the park – we knew what sold and what didn't – and since we were never asked to keep an inventory, there was no way of establishing if a book had gone missing. Once we had perfected our system, we were able to cream off roughly $150 each a week, thereby doubling our salaries.

At the same time, ironically, the management was delighted with our performance, since we were making so much money for the store – more than anyone had made in previous years. The fact that we were foreign, and spoke with exotic accents, worked to our advantage – we were popular with bookbuyers – but we took pride in our job as well, and we put a lot into it. For all our swagger, though, we felt vulnerable. Had you observed us for a couple of days, you would have noticed that nobody from the store came by to pick up our daily take.

Equally, you would have realized that we didn't leave it in the kiosk overnight. To anyone watching, then, it would have been obvious that when we walked to the corner of Sixth Avenue and 41st Street at the end of the working day and caught the subway to Union Square, we had the money on us. Even given the amount we were creaming off, we would generally clear at least $1,000 a day, and that was a lot of cash to be carrying about. Muggings were common in Times Square. We might be seriously hurt – or even killed. Not only were we being paid a pittance, but we were also being put at risk, and the management didn't seem to realize. We began to think of the money we were skimming as danger money. We deserved it for getting on the subway every night. We'd *earned* it.

Remarkably enough, nothing ever happened, and when it was time for me to leave for Tokyo, where I had planned to spend a few months, I was sorry to go. The life of the park had become my life; I would miss the rituals, the banter and the small-time notoriety. Klaus and Maritza came to Newark to see me off. We had drinks in the airport. We took pictures. I was on standby that evening, but there were no seats left, and I ended up having to buy a first-class ticket to Los Angeles. I drank champagne all night and hardly slept.

Only about a week after arriving in Japan, I received a postcard from Klaus. He had been given a new colleague in the park – a real asshole, he said. He had decided not to tell the guy about our scam. As a result, he had to cream off double, his share as well as mine, otherwise the average daily take would jump for no apparent reason, and somebody might become suspicious. He was now making an extra $300 a week. He was thinking of moving downtown, maybe to Delancey Street. Getting an apartment of his own. He'd had enough of living with the Venezuelan girl. ■

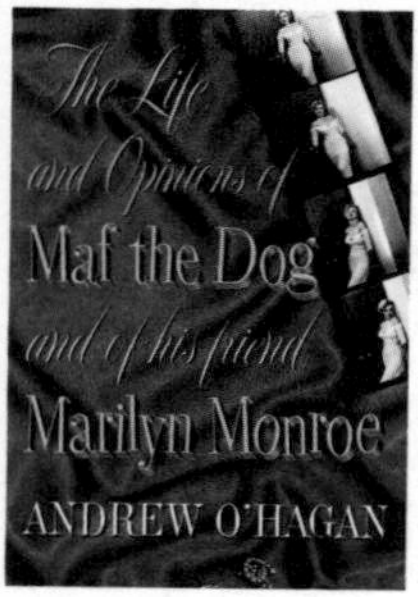

The Life and Opinions of Maf the Dog, and of His Friend Marilyn Monroe *Andrew O'Hagan*

Maf the dog was with Marilyn for the last two years of her life; a real historical figure and the picaresque hero of this hilarious and original novel from the critically acclaimed author of *Be Near Me* and *Personality*. Through the eyes of Maf we're given an insight into the life of Monroe, and a vivid, fascinating take on an extraordinary period of the twentieth century.

Faber & Faber £12.99

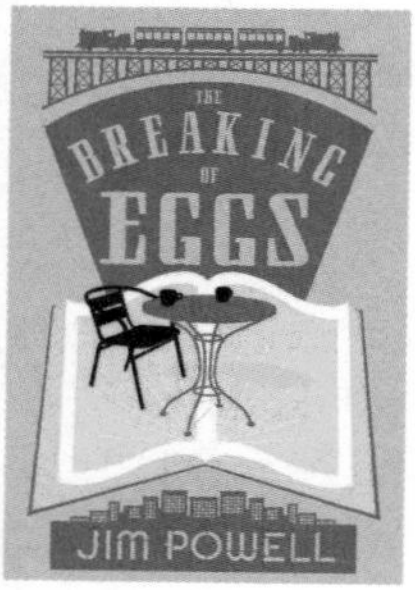

The Breaking of Eggs *Jim Powell*

Feliks Zhukovski is a relic from another age – a man who chose politics over people and ideas over love. His life's work is a travel guide to the old Eastern bloc, but now Communism has collapsed and his travel-writing days are numbered. After fifty years of misunderstandings and delusions, can he start life afresh? An extraordinary and thought-provoking story told with humour and uplifting power.

Weidenfeld & Nicolson £12.99

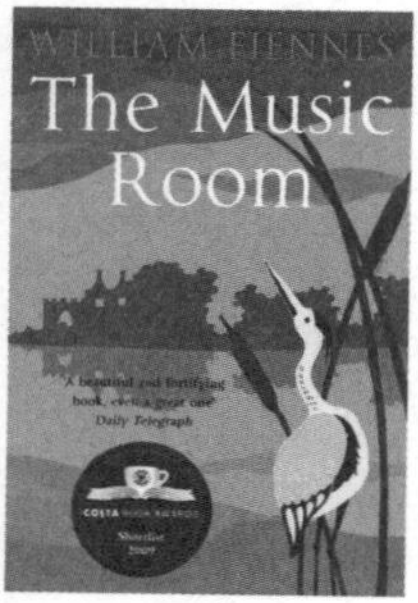

The Music Room *William Fiennes*

William Fiennes's childhood was one of imagination and curiosity. His older brother, Richard, who suffered from severe epilepsy, was an adored figure in his life. Eager to understand his brother's mind, Fiennes has written a profoundly moving account of his home, his family, and above all, Richard.

Described by the *Telegraph* as a 'small masterpiece', *The Music Room* is a luminous testament to the permanence of love.

Picador £14.99

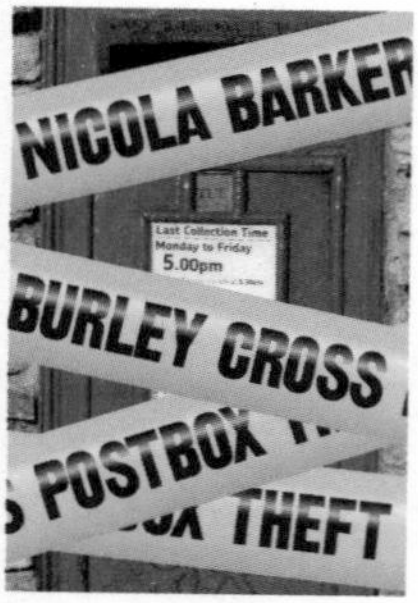

Burley Cross Postbox Theft *Nicola Barker*

From the award-winning author of *Darkmans* comes a comic epistolary novel of startling originality and wit.

Reading other people's letters always provides a guilty pleasure. There's no such joy for two West Yorkshire policemen. They contemplate twenty-seven letters with the task of solving a crime: the shocking attack, just before Christmas, on a postbox in the village of Burley Cross.

4th Estate £17.99

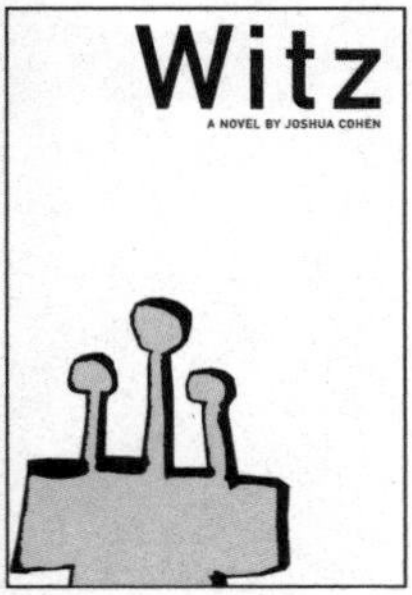

Witz *Joshua Cohen*

'Inspired as it is audacious, three thousand years in the making, *Witz* is the wracked dream of a new Genesis. At the dawn of twenty-first century fiction, the only question is whether Joshua Cohen's novel is the Ark or the Flood.' – Steve Erickson
'An extravagant poeticism combined with an unbridled imagination burst from each considerable page of Cohen's furturistic biblical opus.' – *Publisher's Weekly*

Dalkey Archive Press $18.95

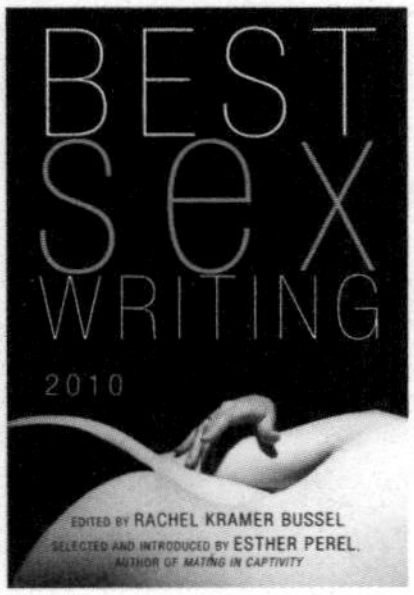

Best Sex Writing 2010 *Rachel Kramer Bussel*

From breastfeeding to swingers to underage sexting, the thinnest condom ever and sex work to the thrill of voyeurism and the story of X-rated Tijuana Bibles, *Best Sex Writing 2010* covers the latest, hottest topics from the world of sex, including the erotic elements of *Twilight*, adult sex ed, a visit to a BDSM porn set, the science behind penis size, and much more.

Cleis Press $14.95

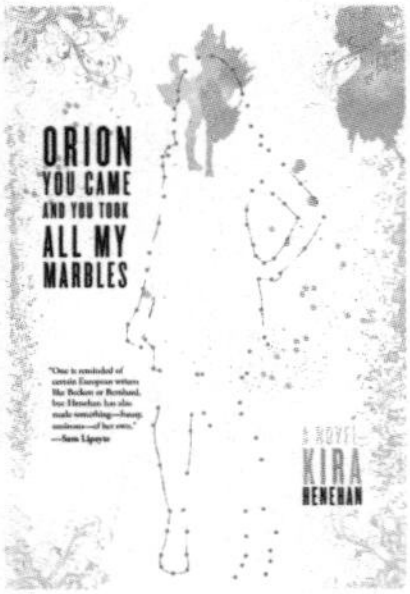

Orion You Came and You Took All My Marbles *Kira Henehan*

Winner of the Milkweed National Fiction Prize.
'A very intriguing novel filled with insistent rhythms and syntactical playfulness. Henehan's precision and obvious delight with language make the voice of this novel wonderful company. One is reminded of certain European writers like Beckett or Bernhard' – Sam Lipsyte.

Milkweed Editions $16.00

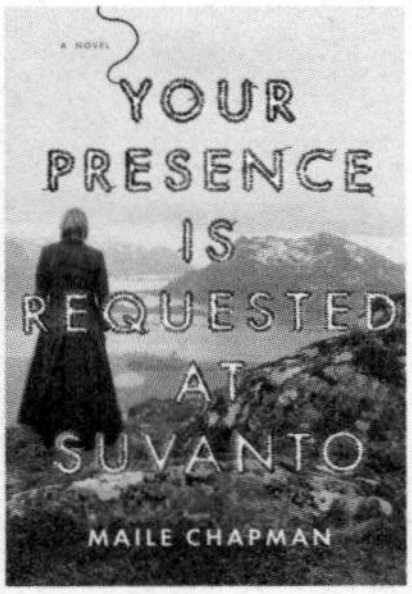

Your Presence is Requested at Suvanto *Maile Chapman*

'In *Your Presence is Requested at Suvanto* Maile Chapman has given us an eerie gift of a novel. It is a superb hallucinatory piercing, an ominous dispatch from that Gothic frontier of the Female Body.' – Junot Díaz
A haunting debut novel about the tangled emotional lives of the mysteriously ill women patients at a remote convalescent hospital in Finland.

Graywolf Press $23.00

STASILA

STORIES FROM BEHIND THE BERL

ANNA FUNDER

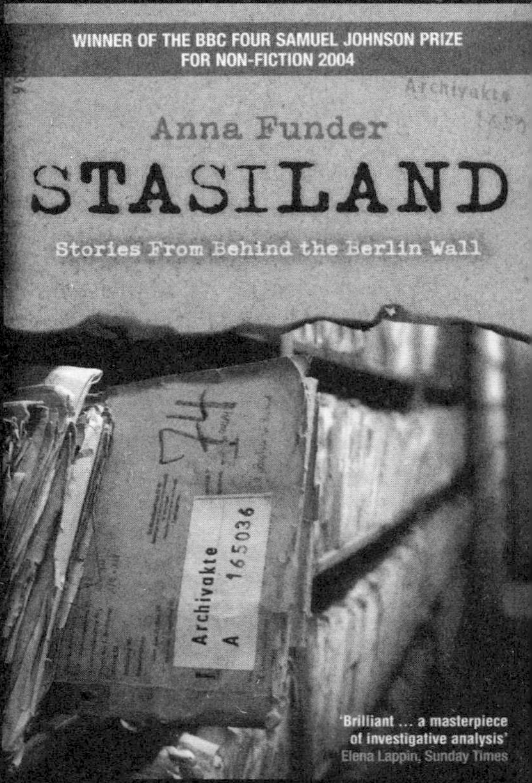
WINNER OF THE BBC FOUR SAMUEL JOHNSON PRIZE
FOR NON-FICTION 2004
Anna Funder
STASILAND
Stories From Behind the Berlin Wall
Archivakte
A 165036
'Brilliant ... a masterpiece of investigative analysis'
Elena Lappin, Sunday Times

'A fascinating book . . . it is written with rare,
I can think of no better introduction to the brut
East German repression' *Sunday Teleg*

WINNER OF THE BBC FOUR SAMUEL JOHNSON PRIZE FOR NON
AND SHORTLISTED FOR THE *GUARDIAN* FIRST BOOK A

THE RULES ARE THE RULES

Adam Foulds

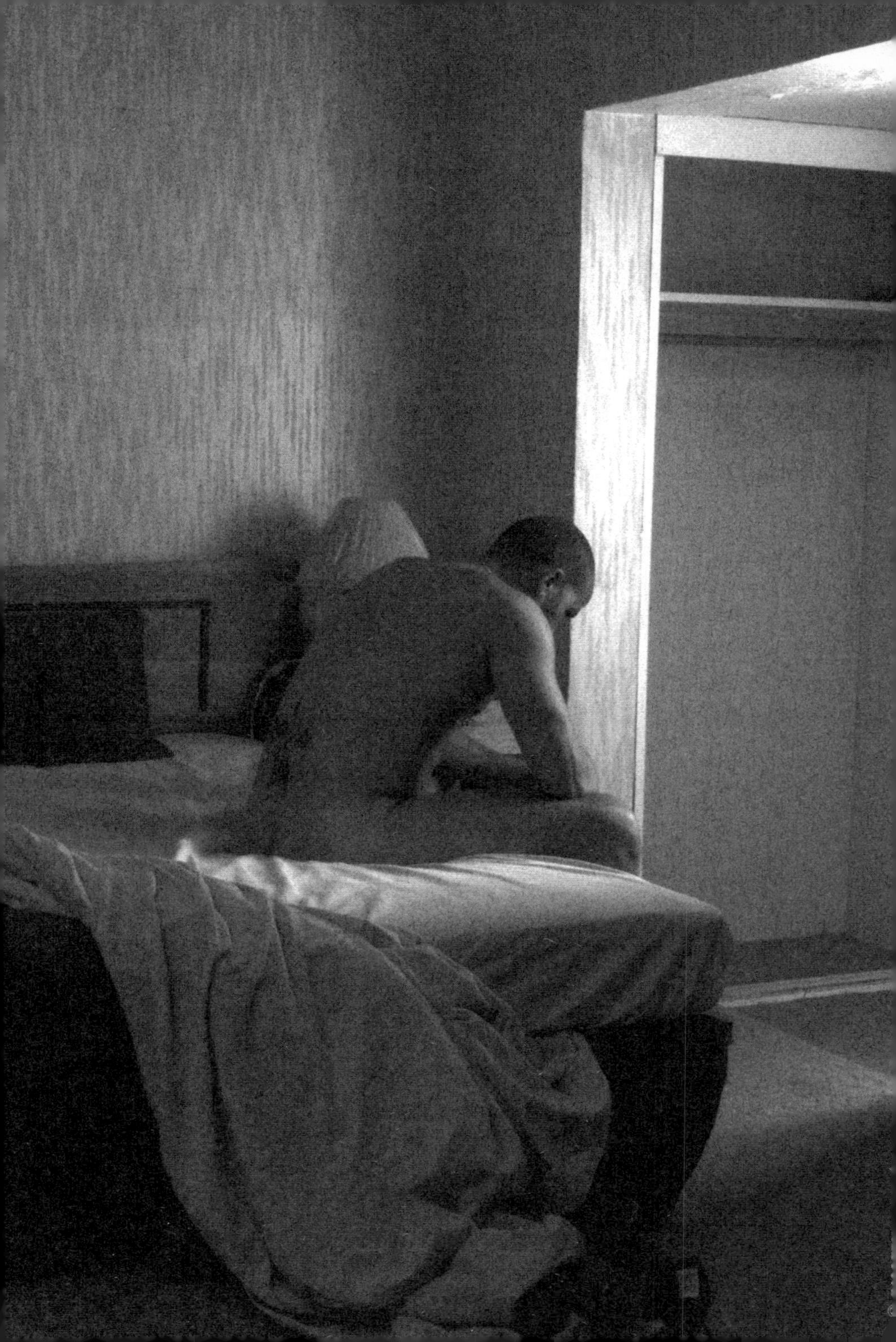

He would have to begin any minute now; everyone else was there: the half-dozen dads on each sideline, the boys shoaling up and down the pitch with a couple of practice balls. They were getting boisterous. He stood up tall and scanned beyond the field of play to the edges of the park. To his left, the low autumn sun shone heavily into his eyes. Elsewhere it made the colours rich, pulled long shadows from the trees. Nothing. Walkers with dogs. Mothers with pushchairs. A cyclist zoomed silently along a path, spokes glittering, and disappeared for an instant behind the back of one of the fathers who held a baby astride his right hip. Maybe eighteen months old. It narrowed its eyes in the breeze, soft hair lifted from its forehead. It held one arm up and tried to grasp with its curling fingers the moving air.

'Rev., are we gonna start?'

'Yes, we are. I was just waiting for Jack. Let's get those balls off the pitch.'

When Reverend Peter blew his whistle he saw a few shoulders in Jack's team drop with disappointment. The boys moved slowly into position. Peter carried the match ball to the spot on his fingertips and just as he placed it, rolling it precisely with his boot, he heard a shout. It was Jack running towards them. He had sprinted ahead of his father whose tiny, bag-carrying form rose and fell far away, laboriously shrugging off the distance.

Peter didn't particularly like Jack. The boy had one of those innocent, insolent faces with an upturned nose and styled brown hair. He was ten and he had a hairstyle. He looked too much like the cinema's idea of a boy, too much like everybody's idea of a boy, and this made him vain. He was vain of his footballing skills in particular. Moreover, he had a professional's tendency to foul, to fake, and to celebrate his goals with excessive displays, running with his arms outstretched, his shirt pulled up over his head to reveal his white, muscled body, his blind mauve nipples. He was strong and pretty and cruel, at least in his careless mastery. Peter's sympathy was elsewhere. It was his natural Christianity perhaps; he felt himself with the boys who weren't as fit or as sure of themselves, the frightened ones. Those boys, however, lit up when Jack joined them.

'You're late.'

'It was traffic. My dad …'

'People are getting annoyed. Just get into position. Right,' he pulled a fifty-pence piece from his pocket and pointed at the opposing captain. 'You.'

'Heads.'

He flipped it up in a spin, swatted it down on to the back of his hand. 'Heads it is.' He raised his arm, blew his whistle and the game began.

The low sun was awkward, flashing uncomfortably whenever the game turned in its direction and heating one side of him. His neck sweated as he ran between the shouting fathers. With sharp blasts of his whistle he cut the game into sections until there was a long period of fluid play when it found its rhythm, the boys in midfield bustling back and forth quietly, the defence lines pulled forwards, pushed back. After minutes of this the boys tired and the game degraded into a series of pointless long kicks, the ball lofted practically from goal mouth to goal mouth. At the end of one run up the pitch, at the end of the tether of his breath, Peter slowed to a standstill. He turned when he heard a baby crying. He saw the child rearing up on its father's hip, its face red and mouth wide. Clear globes of tears stood on its cheeks. Its small fists trembled. The man was doing a poor job of comforting the child. Surely if he spoke soothingly to it and stroked that soft hair it would quieten. Frustrated at his powerlessness to intervene and take the child, he heard another yelp on the pitch, turned again and saw the game halted, a knot of arguing boys around one boy lying flat on his back, rocking from side to side, his forearm over his eyes. Peter blew again and ran over. Blood: a long streak of it down one boy's shin. It poured from a flap of startled white skin just below the knee. Jack was protesting. Of course he was. He reached for his cards. 'Right, you, off.' The boys swarmed around him when he pulled out the red card, tossing their heads and flinging their arms down in despair. Jack shouted at him, 'It wasn't me! It wasn't me!' Peter bent down and asked the injured boy, grave-faced and silent amid the uproar. 'Was it him?' The boy said nothing, nodded. 'Thought so.' He stood up again and felt a brief, cold dizziness of blood draining from his head. He saw Jack's father running on.

'He didn't do it.'

'Off the field.'

'But he didn't.' Jack's father's ears were small, pink and tightly curled. Peter avoided his eyes. 'He didn't.'

'He did do it. The rules are the rules. He's off.'

'You didn't even see it. You were looking at Mike's Janey. I saw you.'

'You and your son, off now.'

'But ...'

'Off. Now!'

He raised the red card for everyone to see and blew as loudly as he could.

The bathroom was warm and heavy from Steve's use, the air scented with shower cream and deodorant and aftershave. Peter arrived trembling from the exercise, his mind marked with the argument. The shower cubicle was warmer and heavier still. A remnant of foam still stood over the plughole, whispering away to nothing. Steve wasn't always very tidy when he was excited to be going out on sermon night. After Peter had showered, watching the soil spiral away, he stood wrapped in a towel, pink and soft, and saw the gunpowder of Steve's beard still in the sink. The lid of his hair gel was off, its contents lashed up into a crest by his delving fingers. Peter dried himself, added his own blasts of deodorant to the funk, then dressed, stabbed the plastic of a ready meal and put it in the microwave.

He ate in front of the television. He told himself it was to find a neat quirk of topicality to add to his sermon, something to remind the congregation that he lived in their world, but he watched quite mindlessly the celebrity dancers in their camp little outfits, taking their turns then awaiting judgement, chests throbbing, smiling crazily, sweating through their make-up. He thought of Steve, perfumed and pristine, sitting on the Tube or already at a bar chatting to someone. Steve, who had arrived like the spring, painfully, changing everything with his provoking warmth, his beauty, who stepped in and out of Peter's cage like it didn't exist, who argued that it didn't exist: *Half the bloody church, Peter.* All that. Steve who was getting bored, who was elsewhere.

Peter felt his rice and meat settling, looked down at his belly. He'd put on black jeans and a black top. Even when he wasn't working, that's what he would put on. He noticed that these two blacks didn't match. The jeans were older than the top; their dye had greyed in the wash. It made him think something, about dailiness, about time spent. The sadness of laundry. Clothes labouring through the wash week after week. *The sadness of laundry! Listen to yourself. Just write your sermon, pray, and go to bed.*

The phone rang, stalling him in his seat. He let it bleat and bleat until the answerphone came on. After his own voice apologizing for his absence: 'Hello, this is Steve …' No, it wasn't. It was the wrong Steve, a non-Steve. 'I'm Jack's father, from football. I thought I'd ring you because I'm not happy, really, with the way things went this afternoon. What you did wasn't … it just wasn't the right call. Jack wasn't guilty and I think you know that, more than you could let on at the time anyway. I sort of wanted to clear the air and just get things straight with you. I've got a very upset lad here and it'd be nice to tell him it'll be all right next time. Maybe you can call –' the machine cut him off with a long beep. In the silence afterwards Peter said out loud, 'Now go away.'

Perhaps he had made his decision quickly and perhaps the evidence had been circumstantial, but a decision had to be made and he was the referee. Also, he'd sensed Jack's guilt; he knew it was there. If he hadn't been guilty at that precise moment, he had been at others and would be again. He was selfish and superb, a greedy player. The boy needed punishing.

Toilet, tooth-brushing, prayers and in. He read for a bit before turning the light out and wondered when he would feel the bed sink under Steve's satisfied weight – alcohol in his bloodstream, semen in his belly – if he would feel it or whether by then he'd be too far gone.

He woke with Steve's arm over him, Steve's mouth against the back of his neck, breathing warmly on to his spine. The back of Steve's hand was blotched with the stamp of a nightclub. He lifted the arm and exited as through a door. Steve rolled on to his back, chewing and murmuring in his sleep.

Peter left early. He liked to be the first person at his church. This was hard to do: his verger, Bill, also liked to be first with his keys, round-shouldered, busy, in possession of the place. Peter walked through a glorious autumn morning. The trees and cars were radiant, their edges haloed with soft sunlight. The fallen leaves were dry, skittering along the pavement in the breeze. Pigeons called from bright aerials, twanging them as they took flight.

St John the Evangelist's was a thick-looking Edwardian church of polychrome brick. It was homely, not beautiful, heavy and earnest and suburban. If he could have chosen his parish church, Peter would have preferred something medieval, something with the ghost of its Catholic past hovering just under the whitewash, something with a hint of the monastic, maybe a preserved anchorite's cell. Still, St John's greeted him with its solid familiarity as he approached.

Someone must have forgotten to put out the sand bucket for the alcoholics last night; the doorway was littered with cigarette butts. He knelt to pick them up. That felt good: a mild abasement. The butts were bent, dingy, sadly human. He filled his left palm with them and unlocked the door. First the bin in the vestry to throw them away, then to wash the ash and odour from his hands. Stepping into the church proper he received the unfailing shock of the sight of the cross over the altar, that jolt delivered by its strong bare shape, by its meaning. He repeated the shape on to his chest with his fingertips, sinking to his knees. In an empty pew at the front of the church, with the noise of occasional cars beyond the glowing windows, he prayed. When Bill arrived, brisk and muttering, a crinkling carrier bag in his hand, banging on the lights, he heard him fall satisfyingly silent out of respect. He gave it a minute more then stood up, smiling. 'Good morning, William.'

His standard Sunday congregation was decent, about forty souls, including the three African ladies who sat in a row under their hats, smiling, and the Davises who sat at the front, either side of young Natalie. She remained placid and bored and pleased with herself, quite still under the arch of her Alice band and long, thoroughly brushed hair. Only her feet swung back and forth impatiently, counting the minutes away.

Peter had honestly tried for a while not to have a church voice but it proved impossible. His normal voice wouldn't carry. To be audible and dignified he needed that slow ceremonial sound. He heard himself go into it at the beginning of the liturgy and it ran like a machine. He could let it function, could feel the motions of his mouth, while up behind his eyes he looked around and thought. It was thus, entering the choreography of the service and delivering solid, meaningful words, that he watched the new couple enter. The man was nervous, tiptoeing with his hands raised, in a pink polo shirt and jacket. He grimaced, baring his teeth as he manoeuvred into place. His wife looked pretty and was, as Peter's mother would have put it, 'in full sail', decidedly pregnant, her face soft and round, tan with make-up. So that was why they were here. They'd be wanting to make use of Reverend Peter's services, arriving late enough in her pregnancy not to have to suffer too much church and soon enough to seem willing. They settled slowly at the back.

Peter spoke and sang. The rhythm of the ritual took hold, appeased him. He saw it take hold of the congregation also. Shaking hands with them at the door afterwards they were clean and light, not quite tired, glazed with smiles as they were let out into the Sunday quiet. The new couple, having watched everything including the exit of all the others, were the last out.

'New faces. I'm delighted you joined us. I'm Reverend Peter.'

The man smiled, but differently to the regulars, as though amused at the thought of meeting a vicar at all, as though this too were part of a show. His fingers were short and heavy, his grip tight. A builder, maybe. His head was set low over high, muscular shoulders. A small gold stud, caught by the sun, shone in one ear lobe.

'Nice to meet you. I'm Rob. This is my wife, Cassie.'

Cassie reached her small hand forwards and smiled with a little scrunch of her nose. 'Lovely to meet you, Vicar.'

'I see you're expecting a happy event, the happiest event.'

'That's right,' Rob replied. 'Fact, that's sort of why we came.'

'Yes, I rather thought it might be.'

'We want to get her started right. And we are local. We live just down by the Peugeot garage.'

'Well, just call the number on the sign and we'll arrange to meet and talk about it. There are things to discuss for a christening.'

'Ah, that's terrific. Thanks, Father.'

'It is, indeed. Another soul saved.'

Rob smiled, his head swaying slightly. 'Exactly.'

Peter watched them walk away. Rob hadn't gone five yards before he pulled a cigarette from his pocket and lit up, his smoke a lovely blue rising over his shoulder.

Peter stretched across the bed to turn the radio down. Rolling on his back he shucked off both shoes and settled his hands behind his head to watch Steve dress.

'I've got a new congregant.'

'Oh yes?'

'Think you'd like him, actually. Terribly butch.'

'Is she now?'

Peter would never mention this, but sometimes Steve reminded him of his grandfather. It was the length and flatness of his back, perhaps stiffening now with middle age. That long plane made his proportions strange when he leaned forwards from his waist to look through the drawer: it was straight all the way up the back of his neck.

'Are you trying to make me jealous?'

'Would I ever do that to you?'

Steve dropped his towel: brief, matter-of-fact nudity, determinedly unarousing. He kept his back to Peter. His buttocks twitched together, hollowing at their sides, when he pulled up his Y-fronts. He sat on the edge of the bed to put on his socks. Now, standing again in his underwear, he looked childish, like a sexy little boy.

'Do you have to go out tonight?'

'And what are you doing?'

'Youth mission.'

'So you're out?'

'I'll be back by nine.'

Steve raised his eyebrows, disbelieving.

'All right, nine thirty. It shouldn't be later than that.'

'Oh, I'm sure. So you want me to sit here and wait for you?'

'You know what I mean.'

Steve chose a shirt from the wardrobe, unbuttoned the top and angled it carefully off the hanger. He slid his arms into it.

'Fine, fine.' Peter gave up. 'Not tonight then. But we should do something one of these nights. I should come with you.'

'No, you shouldn't.'

'What do you mean?'

'Not exactly your scene, dear. And what if someone should see you?'

Peter hadn't apologized because he wasn't wrong so there was no need to. The ball flew high over his head. He always loved that moment, the purity and stillness of it, the ball in another element, silently travelling over the noise below. It sank towards the green. Jack blocked it down with the side of his boot, turned on the spot and looped past the defender. Peter ran towards him, feeling Jack's father's gaze fastened on him. Jack ran three strides and struck the ball cleanly. It shot up, humming, into the top left corner of the goal and Jack stopped still with his arms raised as his teammates rushed towards him. When they'd gone, Peter patted him on the shoulder. Jack turned round startled, shrugged the vicar's hand from his shoulder and ran away. Another boy shouted, 'You taking sides now, ref?' Peter shook his head, back in the game. 'Backchat. Don't make me warn you twice.'

Rob waved as he and Cassie arrived. They sat at the back of the congregation as though still interlopers. Cassie pulled up her bra straps beneath her blouse, settling her heavy breasts. Rob murmured something to her and they both, simultaneously, turned their faces up to Peter. Through the ceremony they were calm and amiable but as if not quite getting the point. They looked continuously expectant, like children awaiting the end of a magic trick that never arrived. Every week they sat like that until they were released into the real world of air and cars and food and TV.

Rob was larger than Peter had remembered. Perhaps he went to the gym. Certainly he had the big cylindrical thighs of a bodybuilder. They held him up on the bulk of himself, as though he couldn't ever properly sit down. Briefly, Peter glanced at his crotch, at his trouser front clogged with his member. Cassie's ringed hand rested on her belly. They looked peaceful, animal, comfortably thoughtless. Rob caught Peter's eye for a hot moment and confused Peter by giving him an inappropriate encouraging nod.

The following week Peter thought that Rob looked hung-over. He sat with his arms folded, his drained grey face tilted back, observing proceedings from under half-closed eyelids. At the door he excused himself. 'Bit dicky today. Must've been the takeaway last night.' He rubbed his stomach to illustrate but Peter wasn't having it.

'I'm sure it was. You can't always trust them, can you? Temperance. Temperance in all things.' That was a foolish choice of word he'd heard himself say twice. Quite probably Rob didn't know what it meant.

He'd chosen the wrong moment to go to the shop. Peter was surrounded by schoolchildren in loud groups. They wandered erratically across the pavement in front of him, shrieking at each other, stepping off into the gutter, oblivious to oncoming cars. Before he could pay for his milk, bread and baked beans, he had to wait behind a few of them as they bought the sugary drinks and sweets that shook their concentration into a useless noisy fizz. He rolled his eyes at the shopkeeper who didn't respond, seemed confused, in fact.

As Peter was leaving the shop, a man entering greeted him. It took Peter a moment to recognize Rob because Rob was wearing a suit. He'd made the standard after-work adjustment: top shirt button undone, tie pulled a little loose. Peter hadn't thought of Rob as someone who would need to wear a suit for work.

'It's Rob, isn't it?'

'That's right.'

Peter often ran into parishioners when he was out and actually quite liked to. It was contact that required only his fluent, professional self, and it made the world sometimes cheerful and friendly, familiar.

'How are you? How's …'

'Cassie?'

'Yes, I was going to say Cassie.'

'She's diamond. Really well. Won't be long now.'

'No, I suppose it can't be.'

'It's a big relief, to be honest, Reverend. Cassie, she, um, she miscarried a couple of times.'

'Oh. Oh, I'm sorry to hear that.'

'Yeah. Well. So. So, we're properly excited.'

'I'm sure you must be.'

'Here, I've got a scan I carry around I can show you.'

'Oh, don't worry.'

'No, no, it's just here.' Rob pulled a folded piece of paper from his wallet and handed it to Peter. 'It's a little girl.'

Peter looked at the faint white swirl, the luminous bones, the brighter white of its heart and spine. 'A little girl, is it?'

'Yes. There.' Rob pointed with the nail of his little finger. 'That blob there is her heart beating away.'

'Yes, I thought it was. You must be very happy.'

'We are. Anyway, I'll let you get on. We're seeing you next week, aren't we, to talk through arrangements?'

'That's right.'

'Great.' Full of his fatherhood, full of his ordinary joy, Rob gave Peter a friendly pat on the shoulder as he left the shop. Peter looked back at him and tried to smile.

Peter walked slowly to football. It was no longer a release for him, a clearing on to which he stepped once a week to move in light and air. Now it was something else that opposed him, another place of solitude without freedom. Dimly he knew that it was his fault, that his personality had seeped out and somehow stained it all.

The day was chilly also, the pitch heavy and stiff. Wind hustled the trees. Cold rain flung across and stopped, started again. The ground was waterlogged near the centre circle. Running through it, the boys' boots stamped up flashes of water that soaked their socks. They played slowly. Jack was impatient, working with more energy and will than the other boys. Peter watched his frustration and indulged the temptation to thwart him further. Three times when Jack had received the ball and was ready to start on one of his glorying flights towards goal, balanced and expert, his hair fetchingly lifted by the wind, Peter blew for offside. It was satisfying to snap the leash and watch him stop, letting the ball roll from his feet, unused. *You're not going anywhere.* He knew he was doing it, that the offsides were marginal at best, and he heard confirming voices of protest from the sidelines. So he wasn't surprised after the game when Jack's father, his face and voice by now so familiar, approached and said, 'Look, I don't know what it is but you've got some sort of a problem.'

'I'm not sure I know what you're talking about.'

'Don't use your posh voice on me. If you don't know, that only makes it worse. I'm not saying you're funny with kids.'

'You better not be. That would be, that would be.'

'I'm not saying that. What I'm saying is that there's something about you and Jack. I've asked him. He said there's no funny business whatever. Point is, I've got a good lad here, a good player, and he's not getting a chance to develop. I've found somewhere else for him, a Sunday league game he can play in. So you won't be seeing us again.'

Peter regarded the man with narrowed eyes, that face so familiar now, the small blue eyes, the sprouting chest hair at his collar. 'I have to say I'm relieved,' he said eventually.

'You what?'

'Jack's a little cheat, isn't he? Can't trust him to play properly at all. It'll be nice to get rid of him. The game will be much improved.'

'Now, listen.' Jack's father jabbed a pointing finger at Peter then shook his head, giving up. 'If you weren't a man of the cloth, seriously …' He turned and walked away.

Off the grid. That was how Peter thought of himself when he lost contact with God, when Jesus was a dead man and he was alone. Then the world was vast and contained nothing, nothing real, only his loneliness between hard surfaces. How long he spent like this was a secret kept between him and God, and of all his secrets this was the most private. Of course this all belonged in the category of 'doubt', which was integral to faith and sounded strong and simple, even heroic, in the spiritual lives of others. But for Peter right now it meant sitting alone in his house with the radio on, the light coming down, leftover baked beans hardening on his plate, and his soul shrivelling inside him like a slug on salt. It meant thinking of Steve out there, loose in the gusty evening city. It meant wanting Steve and Steve not wanting him back.

Sometimes Peter wished for ordinary things, ordinary thoughts. He could have had what the others were having, had he been born that way. But this, apparently, was not what was destined for him.

Peter was angry with loneliness the day Rob and Cassie came to his office to discuss the christening. He sat them down without offering drinks, watched their gazes travel nervously around his bookshelves and religious images, unable to settle.

'You see, this is something to be taken very seriously. Nothing more seriously in fact. Now, I know that I serve a function. I know that's what I do as far as some people are concerned.'

'Sorry, I don't follow.'

Peter stared. 'People need me for this and that, to get their children into the good church schools, to visit the elderly relatives they can't be bothered to see and so on. But I have to insist, I am a servant of God, of Our Lord Jesus Christ, and He demands faith and respect–'

'I understand,' Rob cut in. 'It's a stressful job. You're stressed.'

Cassie rolled forward over her belly. 'Highly strung,' she suggested and lapsed back.

'That's not what I'm saying, actually.'

'And I promise you,' Rob went on, 'we're not taking the mick in any way. We're here – aren't we, Cass? – because we want things done right for our little girl.' Here he reached across and rested his hand lightly on his wife's belly.

'Well, good. That's good.' Peter felt a stab of envy: that was what it was. Recognizing it, his anger gave way. He felt his body soften with contrition, humiliation. He could behave better towards them now he knew. 'That's good. That's what we want to hear. So, I'll take you through the ceremony, what we'll be doing.'

He made them a cup of tea and they talked on. A rain shower rang against the window. It made the room they were in a hushed small shelter. Peter felt close to them. He felt kind.

He walked home under lit street lights and a mildly exhilarating sky of cold silver and long coloured clouds where the sun was setting. Water clucked in the drains. The small trees shone. When he got in and found that Steve wasn't in he didn't pause. He changed his shirt and jacket and went out after him, walking to the station against the flow of returning commuters, tired and grim but still moving at a tough city speed. He sat in an almost empty carriage through the long, rattling journey out of the suburbs and down under the ground.

He emerged in the West End and realized that he hadn't been into town for months. It was dark now. The place was full of entertainments. It had lost its daylight shape and now was structured by its fantasies, by the floating lit signs for different shows and shops, restaurants and bars. The people there all moved towards them or poured away around him down into the station. The traffic was loud. A bus shuddered in front of him. He walked to the street with all the gay bars, to one in particular he knew Steve visited. The street was already full, men everywhere, smoking outside the bars, talking into their phones, laughing, watching. Their hard bodies inside their T-shirts. He passed close to some to get inside once he'd found the place. He could smell them. He kept his gaze low. The music was horribly loud. Its bass thumped right through him like a new and panicking heartbeat, overruling his own. He walked around, couldn't find Steve, and realized he was relieved. What would he have said? He sat at the bar. He could see it all happening from there, could see the desire creeping out between the men. He ordered gin and tonic, wanting to be adult there, wanting to be strict and colonial.

He drank several with a few thoughts beating in his head, like: how different this place must look in the mornings, with the lights on when the cleaners arrive, or: look at that one. The lights in there were strips of blue. Skin looked violet. Cheekbones were sharply shadowed. All this alien beauty. He drank more, expecting Steve finally to walk in. The place filled with more men but Steve did not arrive. Someone materialized next to Peter, a man of about his own age. He wore a white shirt. He looked round at him, at the shape of his shaved head, then let him slide out of view again, but the man put his hand on Peter's. He brought his face close and shouted through the music.

'It's not that terrible, is it? Tell Auntie what's wrong.'

'Nothing's wrong.'

'If you say so. All alone, though. Gloomy.'

'Why do we have to do this?'

'Don't know what you mean.'

'All this. Why do we have to do this?'

'We don't have to, duckie. We like it. I bet you do too.'

'Is that enough? Is that right?'

'Isn't it enough?'

'People don't care. They're not ashamed.'

'Quite right. Absolutely shameless.'

'Your hand's on my thigh.'

'What?'

'Your hand's on my leg.'

'Is that where I left it? Shameless of me.'

'It's not … we don't have to.'

'But we like it. Why don't you come with me a minute? I want to show you something.'

Back at home in the bathroom, Peter took off his shirt, splashed cold water up into his armpits and over his face. He brushed his teeth, rinsed his mouth with mouthwash. He took his clothes off and left them on the floor. He went to bed. Steve was waiting for him.

'Hello,' he said.

'Hello.'

'Where've you been? Blimey, you actually smell of drink.'

Peter pulled the quilt over his shoulder, lay on his side with Steve behind him. 'I went looking for you.'

'I see. Did you find me?'

'No.'

'That's a bit sad. Did you have a good time, though?'

'No. Did you?'

'Not really. Awful, actually. Place is full, everywhere's full of just children really.'

Peter reached behind him and took hold of Steve's wrist, lifted his arm over him, wanting to close that door again.

'Think of you. Out and about.'

'Can't we just go to sleep?'

They weren't there. Natalie's feet ticked back and forth beneath the pew. They were gone, as they had said they would be, to have their baby. Imagine that, the lavish TV drama of it: hospital and pain and beeping monitors, the birth of their baby girl, the tears, the child wrapped in a soft blanket and placed in their trembling hands.

Rob and Cassie had filled the church for the christening. The pews creaked with that laden, seafaring sound that Peter liked. He looked out over the solid formation of their family and friends, the women tanned to varying shades, the men's hair glinting with gel. Rob and Cassie were meek and well behaved, perhaps because they knew Peter's moods and were nervous that all should go well. But for the rest of them, this was a day out, a souvenir experience, and he couldn't reasonably ask more of them. He reminded himself of that and his anger flared during the service only when, with the godparents, they smirked at having to repeat that they rejected the Devil. Christianity: good for horror films, good for a laugh. He stared them down.

The moment that he was waiting for, that he was dreading, arrived. Rob and Cassie's baby, to be named, with surprising good taste, Harriet Sarah, kicking her feet up inside the crisp white cotton of her gown, was placed carefully into his hands. A heaviness swelled in his stomach. It rolled up his spine, flooded his brain. He laid the beautiful small weight of her along his left forearm. Her eyes widened, struggling to focus, as her forehead rolled against his stole. The plush red triangle of her mouth opened as she breathed. The skin of her cheeks was glossy, her eyebrows faint and delicate. A baby. A baby in his arms. The Edwardian font swaying in front of him now seemed dangerously hard and massive. He placed his right hand gently on the soft throb of her belly. To have one, to be a father. He yearned as he stared down at her, feeling sweat run through his thin hair. He glanced up, and the sight of the people standing and waiting shocked the liturgy back into his mind. He said what he had to say. Then, his fingers wet with holy water, he saw a way to disrupt the sweetness of the moment, to release himself. He dipped his fingers again and painted as much water as he could carry on to her head. She looked confused and squirmed against him. He reached for more to apply the horizontal bar of the cross and did so with as heavy a touch as he dared. She rolled her eyes, shrank down into herself then expanded, screaming. Cassie took a step forward.

'Is she all right?'

'What? She's fine. This always happens.' Peter felt sweat trickling down his right side from his armpit, cold at his waist. 'Water's a bit cold.'

'Here, I'll take her.'

'She's fine. She's fine. Please.'

Peter, with difficulty, with clumsy hands, opened his front door, stepped over an ugly splash of pizza leaflets and went and made himself a cup of tea. He put on Radio 3. He took his cup to a chair by the window that he never normally sat in and waited for his pulse to slow. The music was orchestral, late Romantic, with a winding melody that rose to mild crises of percussion and brass. It did have a calming effect sitting there out of place, a little outside of himself, somewhere not soiled with familiarity. The day beyond the window was steady: parked cars, a width of road, the house fronts opposite.

Lying in bed he heard Steve's key in the door, the light metallic scraping. His stale anxiety woke again inside him; it felt as though Steve were fitting his key loosely into Peter's chest, turning him over. He switched on the light and sat up. He heard Steve's tread on the stairs. Then the strong reality of him entering the room – always sudden, always shocking, however long imagined and expected. But this time Steve looked miserable. His shoulders drooped. His gaze was low. He stood as if a bucket of something had been tipped over his head.

'What's wrong?'

'What's wrong?' Steve sighed. He wiped the side of his face as though clearing tears. 'I'm old,' he said. 'I'm too old.'

'Oh, baby. I'm sorry.'

'Course you are. Are you? You shouldn't be.'

'I am. I am. Come here.'

Steve walked over and sat on the edge of the bed. Peter stroked his shoulders, gripped them, swayed him back and forth and pulled him down so that his head lay in his lap.

'Sad old boy. Come here.'

'Hmm.'

'Are you sorry? Are you sorry for what you've done?' Peter took hold of his ear lobe and pulled gently, increasingly.

'Look, if you're going to…' Steve started to get up but Peter pressed down on the side of his head, keeping him there.

'Ow. If you're gonna…'

'Shh. I'm sorry. I won't.' He stroked the soft hair at his temple.

Steve stared, saying nothing, then: 'Course, I'm bloody sorry.'

'Shh. It's all right. Poor old boy. Don't worry. Don't worry. I'm here.'

Peter stroked down Steve's cheek, following the line a razor would take, then over to his mouth, feeling the warm breath from his nostrils. With his forefinger he strummed Steve's lips. Steve didn't resist.

'We're all right, though, aren't we?' ■

SOCIETY OF AUTHORS

The Society of Authors Grants

The Society is offering grants to published authors who need funding to assist in the writing of their next book. Writers of fiction, non-fiction and poetry may apply. The grants are provided by the Authors' Foundation and the K. Blundell Trust.

Closing date: 30 April 2010

Full details from:
website: www.societyofauthors.org
e-mail: info@societyofauthors.org

or send an SAE to:
The Awards Secretary, The Society of Authors,
84 Drayton Gardens,
London SW10 9SB

ROYAL LITERARY FUND

FINANCIAL ASSISTANCE FOR WRITERS

The Royal Literary Fund

Grants and Pensions are available to published authors of several works who are in financial difficulties due to personal or professional setbacks.

Applications are considered in confidence by the General Committee every month.

For further details please contact:
Eileen Gunn, General Secretary
The Royal Literary Fund
3 Johnson's Court,
London EC4A 3EA
Tel 020 7353 7159
e-mail: egunnrlf@globalnet.co.uk
website: www.rlf.org.uk
Registered Charity No 219952

TWO RAVENS PRESS

Two Ravens Press is the most northerly literary publisher in the UK, operating from a 6-acre working croft on a sea-loch in the NW Highlands of Scotland, run by two writers with a passion for language & for books that are non-formulaic & take risks. We publish cutting-edge innovative contemporary fiction, nonfiction & poetry – from internationally acclaimed authors like Alasdair Gray, Alice Thompson & Raymond Federman to talented newcomers. Visit our website to browse our catalogue, read extracts, author interviews, & to purchase books at an average 20% discount with free P&P. Sign up for our monthly e-newsletter, filled with information on our new releases & authors, special offers and giveaways. Read our blog about life as a small literary publisher in the middle of nowhere – or the centre of the universe, depending on your perspective… Feisty, often radical, it's certainly never dull.

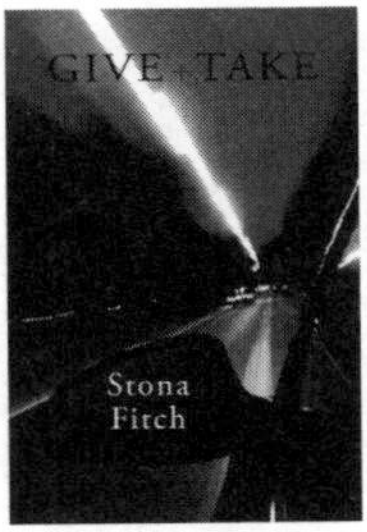

NEW IN APRIL:
Give + Take, by Stona Fitch
'Part noir, part anti-capitalist screed – its voice is both seductive and addictive. A real discovery.' *Richard Price*

TWO RAVENS PRESS

www.tworavenspress.com
We're also on Facebook

POEM | DAVID KIRBY

Psychodynamic Electrohelmet

Fellows, it's happened to us all: you're having
a glass of wine with a beautiful woman at an outdoor
cafe, and the weather's nice, sunny and cool but not too,
and she's wearing this floral-print dress, and one
of the straps keeps sliding down her arm, and she keeps
putting it back on her shoulder but finally
decides just to let it lie there, and you're feeling pretty sexy, pretty

happy about the way things are going and confident
that they're going to get better, when suddenly her eyes
roll up in her head and she says, 'Some people are
doorways to other worlds.' What are you going to do at times
like this other than give credit
to whoever came up with the phrase, 'What are you
going to do?' Why, just the other day, I was putting out the trash,

and my neighbour Richard walks by with his wife, Kim,
and as I'm lowering the bag into the bin, Richard looks
up and says, 'Nice trash,' and I'm thinking, Richard
doesn't know a thing about my trash, and then I realize
he's just making small talk, is trying to be nice himself.
I say there's a lot to be said for niceness,
especially in light of all the stupidity out there: this morning

in the paper, it said that masterpieces are always being
stolen not because there's a Dr No paying top dollar
for Manets and Picassos to hide away on his secret island
but because art thieves think there's a Dr No paying
top euro for Van Goghs and Gauguins to hide away
in his secret castle. The art thieves have
forgotten their Plato, who says, in the *Phaedrus*, that we must

carve nature at its joints, that is, that the world is made
of parts that divide cleanly when we're thinking right,
though when we're not, we're like drunk butchers
swinging blindly at a carcass, our dull choppers bouncing off sinew
and bone. But you can't stop people from having ideas,
especially wrong ones. Where do we go when we leave
this earth? On the shore of tiny Aldeburgh, on the coast

of Suffolk, I saw a war memorial that said, 'They who
this monument commemorate were numbered among
those who, at the call of King and Country, left all
that was dear to them, endured hardship, faced danger,
and finally passed out of the sight of men.'
Where's that, though? In a dream once, I was wearing
my psychodynamic electrohelmet, which is like a 50s football helmet

with a single-bar face mask and an electric cord with a plug
you stick into a wall socket. My psychodynamic electrohelmet
would have explained everything to me, but I never got
to use it. I was at my parents' house even though I was
the age I am now, whereas they were younger than me
even though they're my parents and have themselves passed
from the sight of men. And then I was in France.

And then the dream was out west somewhere, though
    this time I wasn't in it any more, just a lot of cowboys,
        and some had clown noses while others wore tutus.
My psychodynamic electrohelmet would be a miracle
        of rare device, and with it I would build a pleasure dome,
    sunny but with caves of ice, and a beautiful woman
there, and honeydew, and I'd drink the cherry cola of Paradise.

GRANTA

THE AGONY OF INTIMACY

Jeanette Winterson

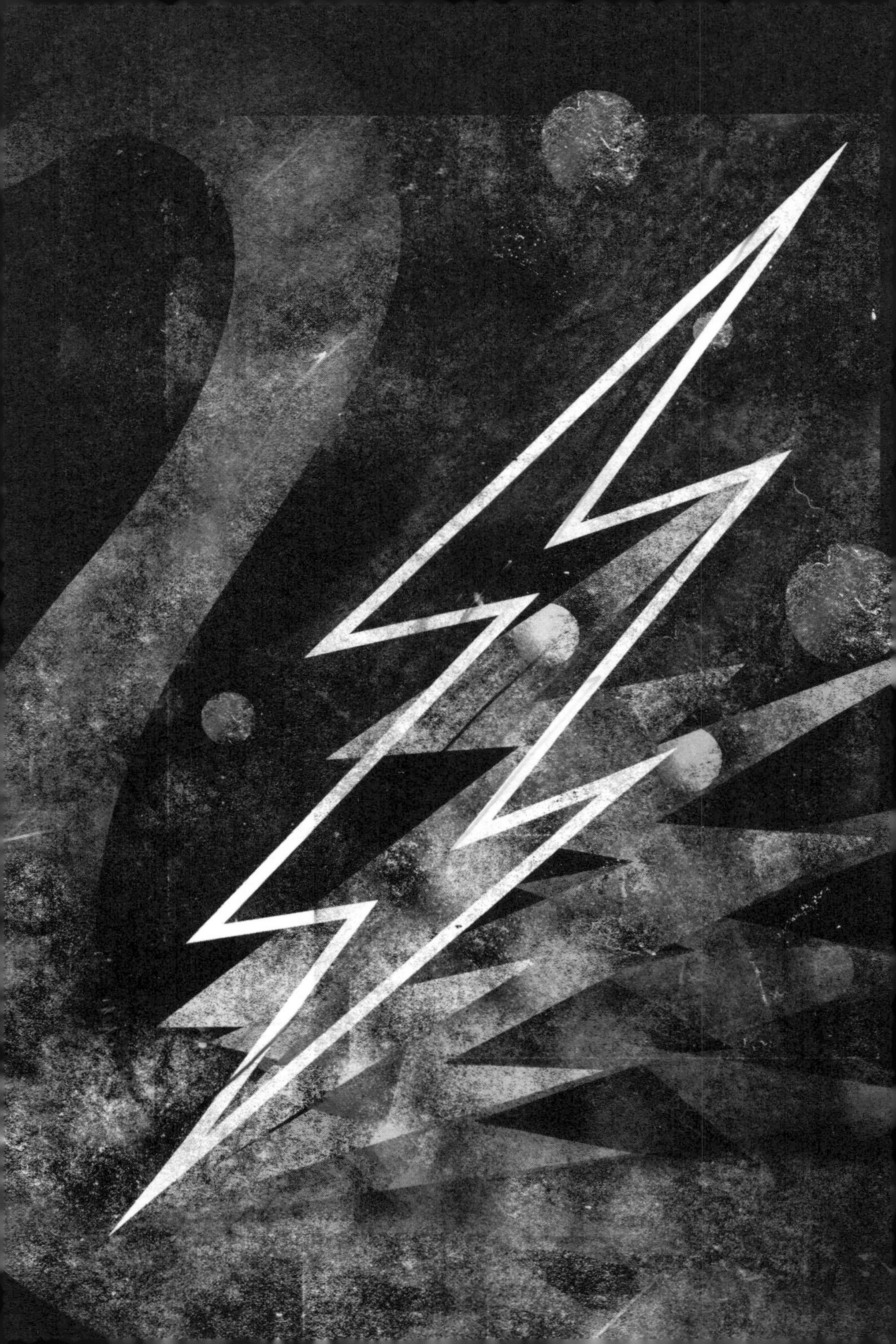

My mother said to me – 'Don't have sex with the gods.'

I said, 'Why not? It's an opportunity for a girl with nothing going for her.'

My mother said, 'Look what happened to Daphne.'

I looked. Anybody who wanted to could see Daphne on the way home from school. She was by the side of the road, green and glossy. She had given Zeus the runaround, ridden in his car, gone to the movies with him, but when it came time for the kisses and the touching, her mother had always told her that good girls didn't do that.

If you wanted to get married and settle down, if you wanted some respect, if you wanted to be true to your sex, sex was not what you did.

So Daphne, who was not doing sex, did the opposite and ran away.

There she goes, her feet in her sandals scuffing the path through the playground where the gods hang out looking for girls. Then she zigzagged into the woods.

Zeus ran after her – he was a pursuer after all, and Daphne should have remembered that. He ran, knowing he could easily catch her, but he didn't hurry, because he wanted the chase, and he wanted her tired, a bit scared, in his arms. He wasn't a bad god, but he was a god.

Daphne was running, thinking about what her mother would say, wondering what would happen if she got pregnant, worrying about school, worrying about money, and everybody knows you can't have sex when you are lying there worrying about everything that isn't sex.

Zeus was not worrying. His prick was so hard it was ahead of him like a dowsing rod. He'd dowse for her. He'd drill her like a well of water, and when she flowed she wouldn't worry any more. She'd spill. She'd be wet.

He wanted her to like him.

This story doesn't have a happy ending.

He was close. She fell. He was on her. She pulled away. He grabbed her. He kissed her. She, in the time it takes to remember, in the time it takes to forget, kissed him. There was a second of surprise. Something happened. Anything might have happened because a world of gas and bubbles and heat was washing between their mouths. Then the known killed the unknown, and he was a god and she was a girl.

It follows that she turned into a tree.

She called for help from the goddess Gaia and her white legs fused so tight no one would ever part them. Her speed slowed. Her arms stretched, her head turned in one shift of yearning. Her smooth skin, wet with sweat, was glossy with plant oil. She tried to speak but spat out a leaf. The lovely rustle of her as she moved in the breeze. Her green eyes were shiny as bay leaves. They were bay leaves. *Laurus nobilis*. She had become a different kind of Daphne.

Zeus pushed himself into the tree of her. She smelled part tree part girl; aromatics and skin. Her leaves still had little hairs from her legs and arms, and where the stem split, where her sex had been, there was sap on his fingers. He licked his fingers. He kissed the leaves. He felt the tree around him, his big confident feet planted at the base of her. She leaned into him and whispered something. It might have been regret.

So on the way home from school when everyone had gone and no one was looking, I went up to Daphne, who'd been dug up and relocated by the school as a warning to the rest of us, and I said, 'Daphne, why did you do it? I mean – why didn't you do it?'

Daphne shuddered in the wind. 'If I had gone with Zeus, nobody would have spoken to me again.'

I said, 'But nobody speaks to you now – you are a bay bush.'

She shook her leaves sadly. 'And I had my future to think about.'

'Flavouring casseroles?'

Daphne leaned her greenness nearer to me. 'He would have left me. He was only after one thing.'

I picked one of her leaves and chewed it.

That night I went for an under-age drink at the Swan. It's run by a woman called Leda who bought it out of her compensation money when she was raped by Zeus. In the old days the gods could get away with it, but now you can call a lawyer on a no-win, no-fee basis.

Leda has tattoos and lives with an ex-model called Helen Troy. A god rammed Helen's mother and Helen, for all her beauty, has a lot of testosterone. She does most of the heavy work at the Swan, and the men who drink here respect her. She doesn't respect them; all that fighting over a piece of tail. She says it was awful being a sex symbol; she would rather have sex – smell, sweat, the agony of intimacy.

She fixed me a cocktail – White Puma – and sat butt sideways on a stool.

'I met Leda in rehab,' she said, 'We were both on drugs – what else is there to be on when you've been multiple-fucked by a swan, as in her case, and blamed for destroying a whole city, as in mine?'

'It was the gods,' I said. 'No one blames you.'

'It's funny,' she said, a short Scotch cupped in her long fingers, 'how we live in a no-fault culture that is also a blame culture. My experience is that the no-fault applies to the men, and the blame applies to the women. But you can't say that post-feminism. And maybe I'm just bitter.'

'You've made a new life,' I say, because I'm of the cliché generation.

'Leda wakes up every night flapping her arms like wings. The judgment was fair – Zeus admitted the swan-work, paid up, went on holiday till the talk died down, and Leda was left to live with it. When you start a new life the past comes with you because there is nowhere else for it to go. One day they'll rent out an island where you can send your past so that it doesn't have to live with you. But until then …'

'Maybe, yeah, you are just bitter,' I say. I don't want to say these stupid things but there's a space in my brain where the complex things should be. I just don't know how to think.

Leda comes over to join us. She is a skinny, white-skinned girl, her pale skin downy, her eyes black like malachite and her white-blonde hair cut short and feathered. She looks like a swan. She slides her long arm round Helen Troy's neck and twists her hand to feel her face. I realize she is blind. I never knew this.

'Swan pecked her eyes out,' explained Helen Troy. 'Judge awarded her 50k per eye.'

'I can see it,' said Leda, 'the swan was beautiful and gentle and strong and still. I was bathing in the river and as I ducked under the water I saw those strong webbed feet parting the current. I saw the green-weed-wet-white underbelly of the swan. I wasn't afraid. Then as my head burst back into the sunshine, the water pouring off me like time, the rest of my life pouring down my shoulders in floods of time, and me standing still in that river of time, not understanding that all my past and all my future had dammed up into this moment and was now pouring out, through, past, over me, so that I would always be in the place and never there again, as all of this happened, and my life was caught in one waterdrop, the swan covered me.

'The swan mounted my back, and anyone who saw must have seen a woman with wings, the great white spread of him out-folded as he used his neck as a noose. His neck made a loop around my neck, his beak hard under my ear, and he lifted me like that out of the water in a beating of wings. The webs of his feet were on each side of me, on my thighs, slightly parting them for grip.

'We rose vertical, then he dropped me on the bank, not letting go, and for a few moments we didn't move at all. A swan's heartbeat is fast. I felt the fast of his heart under my shoulder blades.

'He entered me from behind – not as a swan, as a man, and I enjoyed it. He was slow at first and he had to push and because I was on the ground I let him drive me into the cushiony grass. I was pushing as hard as him because I wanted sex.

'And they never tell you that, the smug people who tell you they told you so ... they never tell you how much you want sex.

'And then I did something stupid. I turned over and I looked at him, as he changed like a trick of the light – swan/man/man/swan. I pulled him into me but I looked at him, and in the looking was the agony of intimacy.

'He reared up. Feathers fell from him. His long soft heavy neck hardened into a cosh. I tried to move. It was too late. No desire now, only fear and rage. Pain. The black beak plucked out each of my eyes and I screamed through my open sockets. He broke my pelvis with the force of his thrust. When they found me the ground was litter-deep in bloodstained feathers.

'They blamed me. You looked at a god, they said, and the gods come in disguise.'

I listened to Leda and Helen Troy. I wondered how anyone finds closeness when violence is so near to it. Maybe the gods come in disguise because they know that – that it is better to take what's there, take what you can, than risk yourself for what will burn you or break you.

Daphne and Leda are the opposite extremes of want – she risked nothing and became less than human. I mean, it's great being a bay tree if that's your lot in your life, but it can't be fun for Daphne. Leda was unlucky – she wanted nothing, and then because she surprised herself into wanting more, she risked everything. She got hurt.

I don't want to be either of them.

Helen Troy was too beautiful. The kind of woman men want so much that they destroy everything just trying to rid themselves of the way they feel. When you feel a lot it's so scary you want to smash up. If you are a man, it is easier to smash something on the outside than it is to feel what's happening inside. Women know it's inside, and so that's what they smash. They smash themselves.

Me, I don't want to smash up, but I don't want to be smashed either. Everyone I meet is really saying the same useless stuff. They say, *Love is everything, throw yourself off the cliff for him.* They say, *Love doesn't exist. Get the money and the house.*

The lovers all die of betrayal and a broken heart. The non-lovers live longer and hate everyone.

Is that all there is?

I said to Helen Troy, 'You should dig up Daphne and re-root her here.'

Helen said, 'That's a nice idea. She could go in a lead pot by the door, then at least she'd have company. No one wants to be alone.'

'Should'a thought of that before she turned herself into a tree,' said Leda, who believes she has suffered more than anyone.

But Helen had gone for a spade, and she told me I could get a ride home in her truck. I got in. I liked the old red leather seats, ripped in places like wounds that don't mind being wounds.

The sun was setting in flakes and bars. The first stars were coming through the sad singing blues of the sky thick with late-homing birds. The stars looked like hope to me.

If love is going to be done differently I will have to do it. I don't mean as a messiah-thing, I mean as a me-thing. I want to look into your eyes and not get blown up. I want you to see me as I am and not destroy me. I don't want to retreat into plant life, or have the same bad dream every night. I don't want to watch a city burn because I was there.

'You're just a kid,' says Helen Troy, glancing at me as she tunes the radio. 'A romantic kid.'

She wants to be kind and she slips her arm round me along the bench seat of the truck. I'd like her to touch me. I want sex. They don't tell you that … I shift myself to get a better feel from the diesel throb of the unsprung truck. I like the feel of everything, just now, tonight. I feel hope like the stars.

I must have fallen asleep because when I opened my eyes I was lying on my back on the seat and outside I could hear a spade digging in the ground. I lay still, listening, thinking. Now the stars were very bright through the glass.

I unzipped my jeans and crooked my knees, my hand moving easily to the rhythm of the spade. A shooting star could lodge in me now and in nine months I'll have a baby I can throw back into the sky the way that happens to the kids of the gods. My shining son will be a reminder of what I did, but I won't regret it. And I think that is the only clue; don't regret it.

Love me let me love you come near me get inside me carry me let me carry you risk it risk everything the stars have been travelling this light all this time let you lie on your back legs open and see it really see it so that it touches you. Touch me.

The star-shot world of the gods. ■

CONTRIBUTORS

Roberto Bolaño (1953–2003) was born in Santiago, Chile. In 2008 he was awarded the National Book Critics Circle Award for Fiction. 'The Redhead' is an excerpt from his novel *Antwerp*, published in 2010 (Picador/New Directions).

Philip Boehm has translated numerous works from the German and Polish and is the recipient of awards from the UK Society of Authors and the National Endowment for the Arts.

Jo Broughton trained at the Royal College of Art and is a documentary photographer and artist based in London.

Emmanuel Carrère is the author of ten books including *The Adversary* (Bloomsbury/Picador). 'This is for You' is an excerpt from *My Life as a Russian Novel*, published in 2010 (Serpent's Tail/Metropolitan).

Anne Carson will publish *Nox* in April 2010 (New Directions) and is currently working (with Bianca Stone) on a graphic novel of Sophocles' *Antigone*.

Brian Chikwava is a London-based Zimbabwean writer. His debut novel, *Harare North*, was published in 2009 (Jonathan Cape).

Linda Coverdale is the recipient of several awards for her translations, including the 2006 Scott Moncrieff Prize and the 2004 International IMPAC Dublin Literary Award.

Marie Darrieussecq has published nine novels, including *Le Pays*, *Zoo* and *Tom est mort* (P.O.L.). Her work is translated in over thirty languages. She lives in Paris.

Mark Doty's most recent book, *Theories and Apparitions* (Jonathan Cape), was shortlisted for the T. S. Eliot Prize. He is writing a prose volume on Walt Whitman, sex, death and the body. He lives in New York City and teaches at Rutgers University.

Jennifer Egan's *The Keep* (Knopf /Abacus) was longlisted for the Orange Prize. Her latest book, *A Visit From the Goon Squad*, (Knopf) will be published in June.

Dave Eggers is the editor of *McSweeney's* and author of six books including *Zeitoun* (McSweeney's) and *What Is the What* (Penguin). He studied painting in college and worked for a time as an illustrator and cartoonist.

Yann Faucher is a London-based photographer. After obtaining a degree in the sciences, he left his native France in 2009.

Adam Foulds is the recipient of the 2008 *Sunday Times* Young Writer of the Year award, the Costa Poetry Prize and the Somerset Maugham Award. His third book, *The Quickening Maze* (Jonathan Cape), was shortlisted for the 2009 Man Booker Prize.

Philip Gabriel is Professor of Japanese Literature at the University of Arizona. He is a recipient of the 2006 PEN/Book-of-the-Month Club Translation Prize.

David Kirby is Professor of English at Florida State University. His recent publications include *The House on Boulevard St.* (Louisiana State University Press), a finalist for the 2007 National Book Award.

Natsuo Kirino is the author of eighteen novels and the recipient of six of Japan's premier literary awards, including the Mystery Writers of Japan Award. Her work has been translated into nineteen languages. She lives in Tokyo.

Emmelene Landon is an Australian-born painter and translator who has lived in France since 1979. She is the author of four books in French.

Victor LaValle is the author of *Slapboxing with Jesus* and *The Ecstatic* (Vintage). His most recent book is *Big Machine* (Spiegel & Grau). He lives in New York City and is at work on a new novel.

Rebecca Lenkiewicz is a London-based playwright. Her latest play is *The Nature of Love* (Faber & Faber).

James Lord (1922–2009) wrote several books (published by Farrar, Straus & Giroux), *Giacometti: A Biography*, nominated for the National Book Critics Circle Award. His memoir, *My Queer War*, is published by FSG this spring.

Tom McCarthy's first novel, *Remainder* (Alma Books/Vintage), has been translated into more than ten languages. 'The Spa' is an excerpt from his novel, *C* (Jonathan Cape/Knopf) forthcoming in 2010.

Herta Müller was born in Romania and now lives in Berlin. The recipient of the 2009 Nobel Prize in Literature, she has also won the European Literature Prize and the International IMPAC Dublin Literary Award. 'Zeppelin' is an excerpt from her novel *Everything I Possess, I Carry with Me* (Portobello/Metropolitan).

Chris Offutt is the author of *Kentucky Straight* (Vintage) and four other books. In 1996, *Granta* selected him as one of twenty Best Young American Novelists.

Carl Phillips is the author of ten volumes of poetry including *Speak Low* (FSG), a finalist for the 2009 National Book Award. A new collection, *Double Shadow*, will be published in 2011. He teaches at Washington University in St Louis, Missouri.

Michael Symmons Roberts has written five poetry collections and two novels (Jonathan Cape). He was awarded the Whitbread Poetry Prize in 2004 for *Corpus*. He is Professor of Poetry at Manchester Metropolitan University.

Rupert Thomson's novels include *Death of a Murderer* (Bloomsbury/Knopf) which was shortlisted for the Costa Novel of the Year Award. His memoir, *This Party's Got To Stop* (Granta), is published in April 2010. He lives in Barcelona.

Natasha Wimmer is the translator of Roberto Bolaño's *The Savage Detectives*, *2666* and *Antwerp*. She is currently translating a collection of Bolaño's essays and will translate his novel *The Third Reich*.

C. K. Williams's new collection, *Wait*, is published in May 2010 (FSG), and a prose study, *On Whitman* (Princeton University Press), is published in April. He teaches creative writing at Princeton University.

Jeanette Winterson was one of *Granta*'s Best of Young British Novelists in 1992. She has published eight novels including *The Stone Gods* (Penguin/Harcourt) and is currently at work on a film about Gertrude Stein and Alice B. Toklas.